ONE WEEK LOAN

A fine will be charged if not returned by the date stamped above

ABC OF
BRAINSTEM DEATH

ABC OF
BRAINSTEM DEATH
Second Edition

C PALLIS
Reader Emeritus in Neurology,
Royal Postgraduate Medical School, London

D H HARLEY
Consultant in Anaesthetics and Intensive Care,
Chesterfield and North Derbyshire Royal Hospital, Chesterfield

BMJ
Publishing
Group

© BMJ Publishing Group 1996

1 004702715

First published in 1983
Reprinted 1998
by the BMJ Publishing Group, BMA House, Tavistock Square,
London WC1H 9JR

British Library Cataloguing in Publication Data

A catalogue for this book is available from the
British Library

ISBN 0-7279-0245-8

Typeset by Apek Typesetters Ltd., Nailsea, Bristol
Printed and bound in Great Britain by
Thanet Press Limited, Kent

Contents

Preface to the first edition

by the Editor
British Medical Journal

Few television programmes have angered doctors more than the *Panorama* feature on brain death: "Transplants—are the donors really dead?" (BBC1 13 October 1980), which alleged that patients certified as brain dead sometimes recovered. Screened despite the protests of a delegation representing the Royal Colleges, the BMA, and the Department of Health and Social Security which met Sir Ian Trethowan, then Director General of the BBC, the programme alarmed the public (as shown by a fall in the number of kidneys donated for transplants) and led many doctors to the regrettable conclusion that they would never cooperate with the media again.

Though they did subsequently screen another, more balanced programme on the subject, the BBC never apologised for the mistakes and the attitudes shown in the initial one; indeed, in Mr David Dimbleby's words, "We stand by our programme". Yet all the publicity had failed to find a single example of a patient incorrectly certified as brain dead under the code used in the United Kingdom.

If any good came out of this sorry story, however, it was that doctors began to explore the complexities that lie behind the concept of brainstem death and the United Kingdom code. Dr Christopher Pallis has unrivalled knowledge and experience of discussing this subject and we commissioned him (in a personal capacity) to write a series of articles for the *BMJ* in the "ABC" format. These concentrated on the more practical aspects of diagnosing brainstem death and have been collected into this book—which contains additional material on the wider aspects of the subject, including some of the neurological controversies.

STEPHEN LOCK
January 1983

Preface to the second edition

The first edition of this text appeared in January 1983 as a somewhat belated response to the BBC's *Panorama* programme: "Transplants — are the donors really dead?" (13 October 1980). Much has changed since then.

In 1980 brain death was an issue that only a few physicians in the United Kingdom had studied in any depth. Its cultural implications were largely unexplored. It was not then as widely perceived as it is today that the criteria used to diagnose death on neurological grounds had to be rooted in an explicitly formulated philosophical concept of death and moreover one that would be widely acceptable in a multicultural society.

What was clearly established in the early 1980s was that no patient in apnoeic coma declared brain dead according to the very stringent criteria of the United Kingdom code (outlined in the 1976 and 1979 Memoranda of our Conference of Medical Royal Colleges) had ever regained consciousness or had ever failed to develop asystole within a relatively short time. That fundamental insight remains as valid today as it was 20 years ago — and not only in the United Kingdom but throughout the world.

In 1983 the cardiac prognosis of the brainstem dead was universally appalling. Asystole would occur within hours or days. In a sense this inexorable and overwhelming practical reality impeded the need to address some more fundamental questions. "What did we mean by death?" and "What were the attributes so quintessential to human life that their loss implied that such life has ceased?" And, perhaps more specifically, "by what physiological mechanisms were those particular attributes maintained?" While the cardiac prognosis of the brainstem dead can today be manipulated within a slightly wider range, the key questions remain. This new edition suggests some answers.

We have been concerned at maintaining both feet firmly on clinical grounds as far as diagnosis (and its pitfalls) are concerned. In that perspective this updated text seeks to explore some wider fields. A new chapter is specifically devoted to the brainstem dead person seen as a potential organ donor. There is also reference to parallel discussions currently taking place concerning the related, yet very different, issue of the persistent vegetative state (PVS). And there are comments on the international dimension which the debate on brainstem death has now assumed. This, at present, centres on cultural contexts, legal statutes, recommended practices, and the role of custom (rather than reason) in some of what is still practised or advocated. The debate has certainly been nourished and, hopefully, clarified by a very wide international distribution of the original edition of this book and by translations of the original text into Italian, Portuguese, Spanish, Greek, and Japanese. If the present edition proves as provocative we will be well satisfied.

C A PALLIS
D H HARLEY
November 1995

1   REAPPRAISING DEATH

The need to reappraise death

A dead brain in a body with a still beating heart is one of the more macabre products of modern technology. During the past 40 years techniques have developed that can artificially maintain ventilation (through resort to ever more sophisticated equipment), circulation (by the use of pressor amines), appropriate nutrition (by the intravenous route), and elimination of waste products of metabolism (by dialysis) in a body whose brain has irreversibly ceased to function. Such cases began to appear in all countries as their intensive care facilities reached a certain standard. What we do when confronted with such circumstances raises important questions. Brain death has compelled doctors (and society as a whole) to re-evaluate assumptions that go back for millennia.

Brain death was well described as early as 1959.[1][2] Renal transplantation was then in its infancy, whole body irradiation being the only means of modifying the immune response. It is important to emphasise this because some critics seem to believe that brain death was invented by neurologists, neurosurgeons, anaesthetists, or intensive care specialists to satisfy the demands of transplant surgeons. If transplantation were superseded tomorrow by better methods of treating end stage organ failure, well run intensive care units would still ensure the production of many brain dead people in many parts of the world.

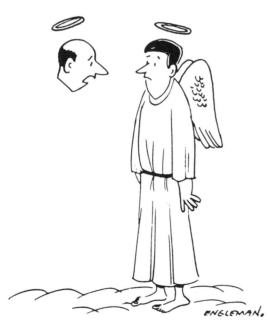

"My brain is dead but they have the rest of my body on a life-support system!"

Over half a million people die in Great Britain each year. Whether at home or in the general wards of hospitals, they "die their own death." No machines or elaborate interventions are involved. Their heart stops, and that is the beginning and end of it. But there is another group of people who have sustained acute, irreparable, structural brain damage as a result of head injury, massive stroke, or very severe cerebral anoxia. The brain damage in question has plunged them into the deepest coma, with permanent loss of the capacity to breathe spontaneously. But prompt action by doctors ensures that ventilation is taken over by a machine before the resulting anoxia can stop the heart. These are the patients — usually all in intensive care units and certainly all on ventilators — that we will be discussing in this book.

We have three objectives: firstly, to emphasise that it is legitimate to equate brain death with death (this is now widely accepted in medical and legal circles in nearly all parts of the world); secondly, to suggest that the necessary and sufficient component of brain death is death of the brainstem (this is less widely accepted, largely because it is a relatively new concept); and, thirdly, to explain how a dead brainstem can reliably be diagnosed at the bedside.

The acceptance of these ideas would lessen human distress, lead to more rational use of our limited intensive care facilities, and radically alter the life expectancy of thousands of patients with end stage organ failure. It would also require that we change the words we use and start speaking systematically of *brainstem death* if that is what we mean.

Mechanisms of death

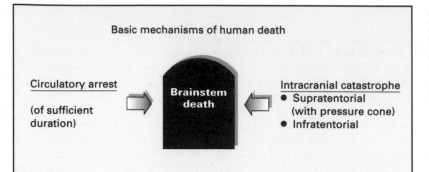

Basic mechanisms of human death

Circulatory arrest

(of sufficient duration)

→ **Brainstem death** ←

Intracranial catastrophe
- Supratentorial (with pressure cone)
- Infratentorial

Circulatory arrest is the commonest cause of death, but it will cause death only if it persists long enough for the brainstem to die. Arrest of briefer duration may result in severe anoxic encephalopathy without critically affecting brainstem function. Such a patient will probably be severely brain damaged, perhaps even in a persistent vegetative state (PVS), but the patient will not be apnoeic (because he or she will still have a functioning brainstem). Sudden failure of cardiac output which lasts only a matter of seconds may cause syncope. In circulatory disturbances of even briefer duration there will be no neurological repercussions whatever. Of all the intracranial neural structures the brainstem seems to be the most resistant to anoxia.

Irreversible damage to the brainstem (causing irreversible loss of the capacity for consciousness and irreversible apnoea) does not result only from circulatory arrest. It can also arise from primary intracranial lesions. In nearly all cases these are supratentorial and damage the brainstem by causing uncal herniation and tentorial pressure cones. This often arises when the pressure in the supratentorial compartment of the cranial cavity is very high. In such cases the intracranial pressure may in fact be so high that the whole cerebral circulation is "blocked."

The brainstem may also be irreversibly damaged by primary brainstem lesions, but this is rare.

There are two basic mechanisms of human death. These will be discussed in further detail in the following pages. We will argue that whereas there are several ways of dying, there is only one kind of death – the death of the brainstem.

Three main areas of confusion need to be studied before we can discuss the clinical problems involved in identifying a dead brainstem in patients on ventilators who have sustained sudden massive intracranial lesions but whose hearts have been kept beating.

Three areas of confusion

- Need for criteria of death to be related to concepts of death
- Death: an event or a process?
- Whole brain death, persistent vegetative state, and death of the brainstem

Concepts and criteria

All talk of the criteria of death—and thereby all arguments about better criteria—must be related to some overall concept of what death means. When we consider death, the tests we carry out and the decisions we make should be logically derived from explicitly stated conceptual and philosophical premises. There can be no free-floating criteria, unrelated to such premises. The box lists several concepts that have prevailed from time to time or that are currently being discussed.

Concepts

- Entering certain monastic orders in the Middle Ages
- The soul leaving the body
- "Ashes to ashes; dust to dust"
- Irreversible loss of the capacity for consciousness and of the capacity to breathe
- Loss of personal identity (the "higher brain" formulation)

Esoteric concepts

In the Middle Ages, if one entered certain monastic orders one ceased to enjoy the limited rights and heavy obligations of the outside world. One would be deemed "dead" by civil society. The appropriate criterion for such a concept of death would presumably be a certificate from the father superior of the monastery confirming that one had entered it. Esoteric concepts would be met by esoteric criteria.

The departure of the soul from the body

The identification of death with the departure of the soul from the body was central to ancient Egyptian culture. It then formed the basis of both Hellenic and Judeo-Christian concepts of death and eventually of the Islamic concept. It would, however, be impossible to derive criteria of death from this concept because of the impossibility of ascertaining the anatomical locus of the "soul."[3] In 1957 Pope Pius XII, speaking to an international congress of anaesthetists, raised the question of whether one should "continue the resuscitation process despite the fact that the soul may already have left the body."[4] The determination of when that had occurred was left for physicians to decide.

Death (irreversible loss of function) of the whole organism

Some people have held that the surest notion of death is the biblical one: "Ashes to ashes, dust to dust." The appropriate criterion for such a concept would be putrefaction, but no one today would argue that this is necessary before a person can be pronounced dead. We all readily grasp the difference between "is this woman dead?" and "has every enzyme stopped working, in every cell of her body?" The controversy is between those who think of death as "dissolution of the organism as a whole" and those who insist that it can mean only the "dissolution of the whole organism". This is no philological quibble. It is well established that different tissues die (that is, irreversibly cease to function) at different rates after asystole.

Asked what they mean by death, most people will probably talk about the heart "having stopped for good". This is by far the commonest mechanism of death (and, until relatively recently, it was also a universal attribute of a cadaver). But is it really a concept of death? When asked whether a person is dead whose cardiac function has, for a while, been taken over by a machine, many people begin to realise that a beating heart is not an end in itself but a means to another end: the perfusion of the brain with oxygenated blood. This centrality of the brain has been unconsciously perceived by people with little or no knowledge of physiology: we have been hanging and decapitating for centuries.

Irreversible loss of the capacity for consciousness plus irreversible loss of the capacity to breathe

We consider human death to be a state in which there is irreversible loss of the capacity for consciousness combined with irreversible loss of the capacity to breathe spontaneously (and hence to maintain a spontaneous heart beat). Alone, neither would be sufficient. Both are essentially brainstem functions (predominantly represented, incidentally, at different ends of the brainstem). The concept is, admittedly, a hybrid one, expressing philosophical, cultural, and physiological concerns. The loss of the capacity for consciousness can be thought of as a reformulation (in terms of modern neurophysiology) of the older cultural concept of the departure of the "conscious soul" from the body. In the same perspective, irreversible apnoea can also be thought of as the permanent loss of "the breath of life." This approach corresponds perhaps to an intermediate stage of current concerns, seeking to maintain a footing on both types of ground. Although seldom explicitly formulated, this view of death is, we believe, widely shared in the West. It is the implicit basis for British practice in diagnosing "brainstem death."

"Cognitive death" and other "higher brain" formulations

Some people, particularly in the United States, have gone further and proposed a concept of death that would equate it with the loss of personal identity or with the "irreversible loss of that which is essentially significant to the nature of man."[5] "Cognitive death" is already being evaluated as part of the "next generation of problems."[6] We are opposed to "higher brain" formulations of death because we fear they are the first step along a slippery slope. If one starts equating the loss of higher functions with death, then which higher functions? Damage to one hemisphere or to both? If to one hemisphere, to the "verbalising" dominant one or to the "attentive" non-dominant one? One soon starts arguing frontal versus parietal lobes.

Over the past 100 years people have sought to "secularise their philosophical understanding of their nature" and have sought to find "more biological formulations of what it meant to be dead."[7] When we strike these existential chords, however, the responses are likely to be implicitly philosophical. If we understand this, we will be more tolerant of the diversity of answers people will give when asked, "What is it that is so central to your humanity that when you lose it you are dead?"

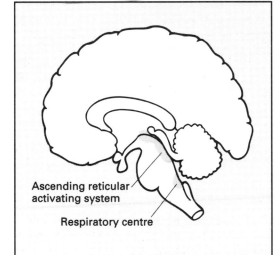

Site of lesions capable of causing, respectively, "irreversible loss of the capacity for consciousness" and "irreversible loss of the capacity to breathe spontaneously."

Ascending reticular activating system

Respiratory centre

Death: an event or a process?

In 1968 the 22nd World Medical Assembly in Sydney stated: "Death is a gradual process at the cellular level, with tissues varying in their ability to withstand deprivation of oxygen. But clinical interest lies not in the state of preservation of isolated cells but in the fate of a person. Here the point of death of the different cells and organs is not so important as the certainty that the process has become irreversible, whatever techniques of resuscitation may be employed."[8] In thus defining death the delegates in Sydney were endorsing — whether they knew it or not — one of the options offered by the *Concise Oxford Dictionary*, which describes death both as "dying" (a process) and "being dead" (a state).

It has, of course, been thought for centuries that growth of the hair and nails continues after the heart has stopped. Surgeons discovered years ago that they could harvest skin 24 hours after irreversible asystole and transplant it. A bone graft or an arterial graft would "take" even if the tissue had been collected 48 hours after death. In the light of such observations the classic signs of death (permanent cessation of breathing and of the heartbeat) will be perceived rather differently: they will be seen as major and easily detectable events, triggering a final, rapid sequence of biological changes. They are the usual points of no return in the dissolution of the organism as a whole and proof positive that the process leading to death of the whole organism has indeed become irreversible.

Legal constraints and dictionary definitions have probably delayed acceptance of the notion of death as a process. A quarter of a century ago an editorial in a leading American journal talked of the "end point" of existence "which ought to be as clear and sharp as in a chemical titration."[9] In fact the simultaneous destruction of all tissues — death as an event — is rare indeed. The sudden carbonisation of the whole body by a nuclear explosion is the only example that readily comes to mind.

In the heat of the public controversy about brain death in 1981 a limerick was written which summed up the simple wisdom that death is a process:

> In our graveyards with winter winds blowing
> There's a great deal of to-ing and fro-ing
> But can it be said
> That the buried are dead
> When their nails and their hair are still growing?

We think all cultures capable of asking such a question would answer it with an unequivocal "yes" whether the premises were true or not.

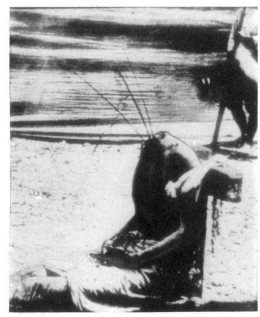

Anatomical decapitation. Heart is still beating as shown by jets of blood from carotid and vertebral arteries.

There are other points of no return. One type of event epitomises the fact that death may precede cessation of the heart beat: decapitation. Once the head has been severed from the neck the heart continues to beat for up to an hour.[10] Is that person alive or dead? If those who hold that a person can be truly dead only when the heart has stopped believe that a decapitated person is still alive simply because parts of the heart are still beating, they have a concept of life so different from ours that we doubt if bridges could be built. The example given is one of *anatomical* decapitation. Brain death is *physiological* decapitation and usually occurs when the intracranial pressure has lastingly exceeded the arterial pressure. Nevertheless, the implications of the two types of decapitation are similar. They are that the death of the brain is the necessary and sufficient condition for the death of the individual person.

The persistent vegetative state, whole brain death, and death of the brainstem

About 25 years ago a picture of an unsuccessfully decapitated chicken appeared in a leading magazine. The forebrain had been amputated and lay on the ground. The brainstem was still in situ. The animal, still breathing, was photographed some time after the decapitation. Was it alive or dead?

In our opinion the animal must be considered alive so long as its brainstem is functioning. Let us extrapolate the argument to a child with hydranencephaly. There is a spinal cord, a brainstem, and perhaps some diencephalic structures but certainly no cerebral hemispheres. The cranial cavity is full of cerebrospinal fluid, transilluminates when a light is applied to it, and there is no detectable electroencephalographic activity. The child can breathe spontaneously, swallow, and grimace in response to painful stimuli. Its eyes are open. The heart can beat normally for many weeks. No culture would declare that child dead. This emphasises the centrality we instinctively allocate to persisting brainstem function, even in the absence of anything we could describe as cerebration.

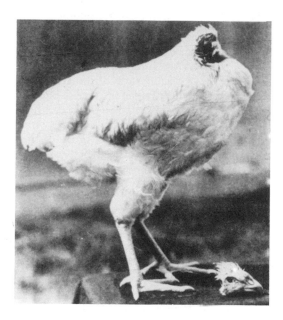

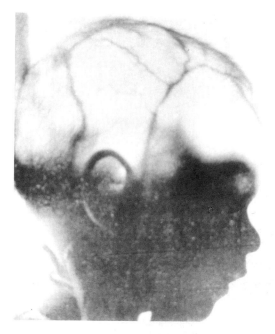

These examples may help one grasp the essence of a much more common and important condition: the persistent vegetative state. This is a chronic condition, the result of either cerebral anoxia (which may devastate the cortical mantle of the brain) or of impact injury to the head (which may massively shear the subcortical white matter, disconnecting the cortex from underlying structures). Other pathological processes may also on occasion be responsible. Affected people, if adequately nursed, may survive for years. They open their eyes so that by definition they cannot be described as comatose. But, although awake, they show no behavioural evidence of awareness. Conjugate roving movements of the eye are common, orientating movements rare. The patients do not speak or initiate purposeful movement of their limbs. Abnormal motor responses to stimulation may often be seen. Like the hydranencephalic child, the patients grimace, swallow, and breathe spontaneously. Their pupillary and corneal reflexes are usually preserved. They have a working brainstem but show no evidence of meaningful function above the level of the tentorium. Excellent reviews of the pathological basis of the persistent vegetative state[11] and of the difficulties in determining its limits[12] have been recently published.

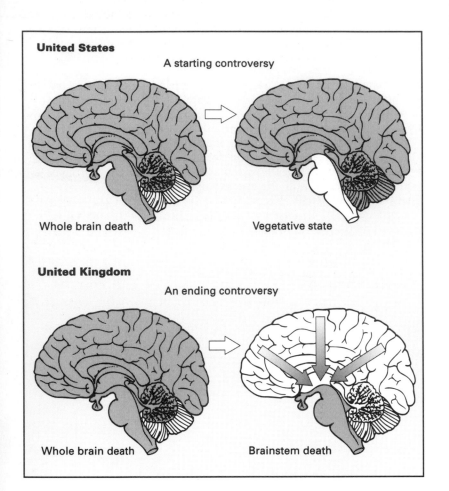

United States

A starting controversy

Whole brain death → Vegetative state

United Kingdom

An ending controversy

Whole brain death → Brainstem death

We have described the persistent vegetative state to contrast it with brainstem death. Patients whose brainstems are dead are in deep irreversible coma. They show no sleep–wake sequences. Their brainstem reflexes cannot be elicited. They have irreversibly lost the capacity to breathe. Brainstem death is the physiological kernel of brain death, the anatomical substratum of its cardinal signs (apnoeic coma with absent brainstem reflexes), and the main determinant of its invariable cardiac prognosis: inevitable asystole.

The illustration shows the controversy which has developed in the United States between the vast majority who have accepted death as synonymous with "death of all structures above the foramen magnum" (so called "whole brain death") and others, mainly philosophers, suggesting that death of large parts of both cerebral hemispheres ("neocortical death," "cognitive death," "persistent vegetative state") might itself be enough to consider a patient dead. It also shows the shift of emphasis that has occurred in the United Kingdom from a concept of brain death as a state in which "all functions of the brain have permanently and irreversibly ceased" to another in which the brainstem is perceived as "the critical system of the critical system" and in which "permanent functional loss of the brainstem constitutes brain death."

Another controversy centres on whether physicians can identify death of the brainstem by exclusively clinical (non-instrumental) methods and about what flows from such an identification. When people engaged in one discussion are suddenly parachuted into one of the others communication is bound, for a while, to be difficult.

Determining death and "allowing to die"

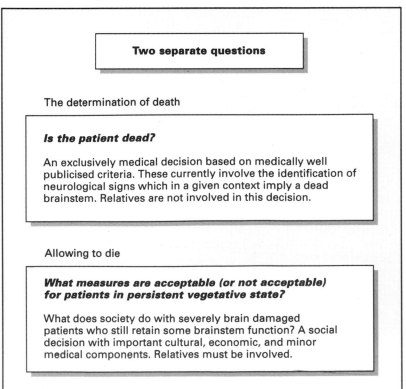

Two separate questions

The determination of death

Is the patient dead?

An exclusively medical decision based on medically well publicised criteria. These currently involve the identification of neurological signs which in a given context imply a dead brainstem. Relatives are not involved in this decision.

Allowing to die

What measures are acceptable (or not acceptable) for patients in persistent vegetative state?

What does society do with severely brain damaged patients who still retain some brainstem function? A social decision with important cultural, economic, and minor medical components. Relatives must be involved.

Two further questions tend to get muddled when people talk about death. The first is the determination of death: Is the patient dead? This should be a medical decision based on medically defined, clearly formulated, and well publicised criteria. The current problem is the recognition of a constellation of neurological signs which we can equate with irreversible loss of brainstem function. To say that the answer should be medical does not mean that society, through its laws, should not seek to reflect public opinion and outline an acceptable conceptual framework within which its doctors can work.

Discussions about "allowing to die" are different. They seek to answer very difficult questions about how society copes with severely brain damaged patients who still have some brainstem function (the Karen Quinlan dilemma).

There are patients of this kind in long term care units all over the world. They are an enormous social problem. Decisions have to be taken about them. But these are social decisions with important cultural, ethical, religious, and economic implications. There are medical implications too, but doctors should not try to play God; their function is to give an early prognosis (if they can). There have been important advances in this subject.[13][14] The whole issue has been extensively reviewed in a House of Lords' report.[15] Different societies at different times have taken different attitudes to this problem, which abuts on to the whole subject of passive euthanasia. But we are not discussing euthanasia. "The uncomfortable dimensions of the care of the dying"[16] have nothing to do with identifying a dead brainstem.

1 Wertheimer P, Jouvet M, Descotes J. A propos du diagnostic de la mort du système nerveux dans le comas avec arrêt respiratoire traités par la respiration artificielle. *Presse Med* 1959; **67**:87–8.
2 Mollaret P, Goulon M. Le coma dépassé (mémoire préliminaire). *Rev Neurol (Paris)* 1959; **101**:3–15
3 Corner GW. Anatomists in search of the soul. *Ann Med Hist* 1919; 2:1–7.
4 Pius XII, Pope. Prolongation of life. *Pope Speaks* 1957; 4:393–8.
5 Veatch RM. Brain death: welcome definition or dangerous judgment. *Hastings Center Report* 1972; ii:10–13.
6 Beresford HR. Cognitive death: differential problems and legal overtones. *Ann N Y Acad Sci* 1978; **315**:339–48.
7 Veatch RM. The definition of death: ethical, philosophical, and policy confusion. *Ann N Y Acad Sci* 1978; **315**:307–21.
8 Gilder SSB. Twenty-second World Medical Assembly. *BMJ* 1968; iii:493–4.
9 Anonymous. What and when is death? *JAMA* 1968; **204**:219–20.
10 Dujardin-Beaumetz et Evrard. Note historique et physiologique sur le supplice de la guillotine. *Bulletin de la Société de Medicine Légale de France* 1870; 5:49–74.
11 Kinney HC, Samuels MA. Neuropathology of the persistent vegetative state. A review. *J Neuropath Experim Neurology* 1994; **53**:548–58.
12 Bernat JL. The boundaries of the persistent vegetative state. *J Clin Ethics* 1992; 3:176–80.
13 Levy DE, Bates D, Caronna JJ, *et al.* Prognosis in non-traumatic coma. *Ann Intern Med* 1981; **94**:293–301.
14 Jennett B, Teasdale G, Braakman R, *et al.* Prognosis of patients with severe head injury. *Neurosurgery* 1979; 4:283–8.
15 Select Committee on Medical Ethics Report. London: HMSO, 1994. (HL paper 21–1.)
16 Lewis H P. Machine medicine and its relation to the fatally ill. *JAMA* 1968; **206**:387–8.

The earliest references in the neurological literature to states resembling what would today be called "brain death" go back to the end of the nineteenth century, when Victor Horsley[1] reported that patients suffering from depressed fractures of the skull, cerebral haemorrhage, and brain tumours "die from respiratory and not from cardiac failure, as is often supposed." Clinical observations had led him to conclude that in such cases "the respiration suddenly ceased, the heart continuing to beat." "Such" he wrote, "was the common end of practically all cases of pathological intracranial tension."

Four years later, in 1898, Sir Dyce Duckworth, honorary physician to HRH the Prince of Wales, read a paper (in French) to an international congress in Moscow in which he described "some cases of cerebral disease in which the function of respiration entirely ceases for some hours before that of the circulation."[2] Two of his patients had temporosphenoidal abscesses, one had a cerebellar abscess, and one had a cerebral haemorrhage that had ruptured into the ventricles. All were comatose, and artificial respiration was resorted to in each case. Duckworth commented that "with respiratory cessation death had practically already begun." Harvey Cushing (1902) had finally emphasised the importance of such cases when he wrote "in death from a fatal increase in intracranial tension the arrest of respiration precedes that of the heart . . . prompt surgical relief, with a wide opening of the calvarium, may save life even in desperate cases with pronounced medullary involvement."[3] This early emphasis on the centrality of brainstem function (and in particular of apnoea) and on the importance of excluding reversible causes of such disturbances has a very modern resonance.

Despite these early references to what was probably brain death the condition was only to be described in some detail in 1959 when two French physicians identified a condition they called "coma dépassé" — literally, a state beyond coma.[4] Twenty of their 23 patients were suffering from primary intracranial disorders and the three others from the cerebral effects of cardiorespiratory arrest. All the classic features of brain death are found in this early report. As well as obvious signs indicating death of both brain and spinal cord the authors mentioned poikilothermia, diabetes insipidus, a sustained hypotension which proved increasingly difficult to control with pressor amines, and a progressive acidosis, initially respiratory and later metabolic. Awed by the potential of resuscitatory techniques the authors described the condition created as both "une révélation et une rançon." The revelation related to the capacities of the contemporaneous intensive care technology and the ransom to what the maintenance of patients in this state imposed on others. Those affected were said to have the appearance of "corpses with a good volume pulse."[5]

Articles published in the early 1960s already hinted that the cerebral circulation was "blocked" by raised intracranial pressure in most of these cases. These early publications also suggested the presence of cerebral oedema and intracranial hypertension. Within a few years "blocked" cerebral circulation was to be recognised as a very common concomitant of the condition.

Although major French contributions can be said to have heralded all modern discussions about brain death, it was the 1968 report of the ad hoc committee of Harvard Medical School which brought awareness of brain death to a much wider audience.[6] Possibly influenced by the French, the committee initially used the term "irreversible coma" to describe the brain death syndrome; this has led to untold confusion as the words "irreversible coma" were later to be used to describe a very different clinical entity. A major multicentre project on brain death (the American Collaborative Study — see chapter 9) used the words "irreversible coma" to refer to "a vegetating state in which all functions

Harvard criteria (1968)

- Unreceptive and unresponsive
- No movements (observe for one hour)
- Apnoea (3 minutes off respirator)
- Absence of elicitable reflexes
- Isoelectric electroencephalogram "of great confirmatory value" (at 5 μv/mm)

All the above tests should be repeated at least 24 hours later, and there should be no change

Brainstem death: the first insight

What we are attempting to define and establish beyond reasonable doubt is the state of irreversible damage to the brainstem. It is the point of no return.

Mohandas and Chou[8]

Minnesota criteria (1971)

- Known and irreparable intracranial lesion
- No spontaneous movement
- Apnoea (4 minutes)
- Absent brainstem reflexes
- All findings unchanged for at least 12 hours

Electroencephalography **not** mandatory

The limb reflexes in brainstem death

- The tendon (stretch) reflexes of the limbs are segmental spinal reflexes
- Brainstem death may be complicated by spinal shock causing areflexia
- After an interval if the spinal cord is viable abnormal reflexes will appear below the level of a dead brainstem
- The reflex pattern in the limbs is of no prognostic value in cases of brainstem death

attributed to the cerebrum are lost but certain vital functions such as respiration, temperature, and blood pressure regulation may be retained." This could have been a classic pre-emptive description of the persistent vegetative state. In view of these ambiguities the words "irreversible coma" are best avoided altogether.

The Harvard criteria demanded that the patient should be unreceptive and unresponsive, the most intensely painful stimuli evoking "no vocal or other response, not even a groan, withdrawal of a limb or quickening of respiration" (*sic*). No movements were to occur during observation for one hour. Apnoea was to be confirmed by three minutes off the respirator (the centrality of apnoea, properly defined and tested for, had already been appreciated). The quantification in terms of Paco$_2$ levels reached during disconnection tests came only much later as a result of British experience. The Harvard criteria also required that there should be "no reflexes," the emphasis being on brainstem reflexes. A flat or isoelectric electroencephalogram at high gain was of "great confirmatory value." All the tests were to be repeated at least 24 hours later with no changes in the findings.

The report unambiguously proposed that this clinical state should be accepted as death, recognised the moral, ethical, religious, and legal implications, and boldly saw itself as preparing the way "for better insight into all these matters as well as for better law than is currently applicable." A year later Beecher, the chairman of the Harvard committee, stated that this body was "unanimous in its belief that an electroencephalogram was not essential to a diagnosis of irreversible coma," although it could provide "valuable supporting data."[7]

Within three years of this radical yet humane proposal two neurosurgeons from Minneapolis made the challenging suggestion that "in patients with known but irreparable intracranial lesions" irreversible damage to the brainstem was the "point of no return." The diagnosis "could be based on clinical judgment."[8]

The Minnesota neurosurgeons had introduced the notion of aetiological preconditions. (Twenty of their 25 patients had sustained massive craniocerebral trauma, and the remaining five were suffering from other primary intracranial disorders.) They emphasised the importance of apnoea in the determination of brain death; in fact they insisted on four minutes of disconnection from the respirator. (Alarmingly to us today, they did not mention pre-oxygenation *before* disconnection or diffusion oxygenation *during* the procedure.) They demanded absent brainstem reflexes, stated that the findings should not change for at least 12 hours, and emphasised that the electroencephalogram was not mandatory for the diagnosis. Their recommendations later became known as the Minnesota criteria and were to influence thinking and practice in the United Kingdom considerably. We are emphasising this because it has been suggested that doctors in the United Kingdom have been overcritical of much American work on this subject.

Since 1971 doctors have sought to identify the necessary and sufficient component (or physiological kernel) of brain death. It was soon realised that absent tendon reflexes (deemed essential in both the French and Harvard criteria) really implied loss of function of the spinal cord and that this was irrelevant in a diagnosis of brain death. The original insistence of the French on areflexia is strange for the works of Babinski contain accounts of knee jerks persisting for up to eight minutes after decapitation on the guillotine.[9] Death of the brain and death of the whole nervous system are not the same thing. If the heart beat continues for long enough many patients with dead brains will recover tendon reflexes in the limbs or show pathological limb reflexes.[10] The presence or absence of such reflexes, while providing useful clues as to whether the spinal cord is alive or dead, tell us nothing about whether the brainstem is functioning or not. Spinal areflexia is in fact the exception in brain death (established by the angiographic demonstration of a non-perfused brain).[11]

In retrospect it is interesting that insight into the importance of the brainstem had been achieved as early as 1964, seven years before the publication of the Minnesota criteria when Professor Keith Simpson, asked by the Medical Protection Society for words to use in a test case, suggested that "there is life so long as a circulation of oxygenated blood is maintained to live brainstem centres."[12]

Irreversible loss of brainstem function

> **The basic propositions**
>
> - Irreversible loss of brainstem function is as valid a yardstick of death as cessation of the heart beat
> - The loss of brainstem function can be determined operationally in clinical terms
> - The irreversibility of the loss is determined by:
>   - A context of irremediable structural brain damage
>   - The exclusion of reversible causes of loss of brainstem function (hypothermia, drugs, severe metabolic disturbances)

The box highlights the implications of the memoranda on brain death issued by the Conference of Medical Royal Colleges and their Faculties in the United Kingdom in 1976 and 1979. The first memorandum (which we will call the United Kingdom code) emphasises that "permanent functional death of the brainstem constitutes brain death" and that this should be diagnosed in a defined context (irremediable structural brain damage) and after certain specified conditions have been excluded.[13] It showed how the permanent loss of brainstem function can be determined clinically and describes simple tests for recognising the condition. The second memorandum identified brain death with death itself but did not explain the basis of the identification.[14] These documents mark a milestone in thinking about brain death and have already influenced practice in most English speaking countries and in many others. A more recent report published in 1995 reinforced the previous views and stipulated yet again that instrumental diagnosis was not essential.[15] It defined death as "the irreversible loss of the capacity for consciousness combined with the irreversible loss of the capacity to breathe" and recommended that when death is diagnosed on neurological grounds the condition should be referred to as "brainstem death."

What the proposals imply

> **Two important conceptual steps**
>
> - From classic death ⇒ whole brain death
> - From whole brain death ⇒ brainstem death

Two major conceptual strides are necessary before one can accept the propositions implicit in the Conference memoranda or reports.[13-15] The first is the step from classic death to whole brain death. In most countries medical opinion accepted the basic concept of brain death, although there are still a few influenced by religious or other considerations who oppose it.[16 17] Leading spokespeople of all the main Western religions have endorsed it,[18] and publications on the subject are numerous.[19-21]

Doctors were still taking this first step when they were faced with another challenge: that the brainstem was "the critical system of the critical system" and that death of the brainstem was the necessary and sufficient component of whole brain death. It has already been explained (chapter 1) how death of the brainstem relates to a given philosophical concept of death (the irreversible loss of the capacity for consciousness combined with the irreversible loss of the capacity to breathe). The task is now to convince people that this condition can be identified clinically and that it is not in conflict with more traditional notions of brain death or of death itself.

Some neurologists — and many experts in electroencephalography — have been caught off balance by these essentially conceptual developments. Some of the early and influential proponents of the idea of whole brain death (their first battle won, the role of their electroencephalographs well defined, their skill widely accepted) have proved reluctant to take the second step.

Functions of the brainstem

It has long been known that small, strategically situated lesions of the brainstem of acute onset and affecting the paramedian tegmental area bilaterally cause prolonged coma because they damage critical parts of the ascending reticular activating system.[22 23]

The reticular formation constitutes the central core of the brainstem and projects to wide areas of the limbic system and neocortex. Projections from the upper part of the brainstem are responsible for alerting mechanisms. These can be thought of as generating the *capacity* for consciousness. The *content* of consciousness (what a person knows, thinks, or feels) is a function of activated cerebral hemispheres. But unless there is a functioning brainstem "switching on" the hemispheres one cannot envisage such a content. There is evidence that brainstem injury in humans may massively reduce cerebral oxidative metabolism,[24] cerebral blood flow,[25] or both.[26] Apart from mechanisms essential for respiration the brainstem contains others which contribute to maintaining blood pressure. All the motor outputs from the hemispheres have to travel through the brainstem, as do all the sensory inputs to the brain (other than sight and smell).

Because the brainstem nuclei are so near one another brainstem function can be clinically evaluated in a unique way. Testing the various cranial nerve reflexes probes the brainstem slice by slice as if it were salami. Respiratory function can also be assessed accurately. An acute, massive, and irreversible brainstem lesion (primary or secondary) prevents meaningful functioning of the "brain as a whole," even if groups of nerve cells may for a short while still emit signals of biological activity. The relevance (or irrelevance) of any residual activity above (or below) a dead brainstem should always be related to an overall philosophical concept of death. Those who think such activity important should always be asked to what concept of death they believe it to be relevant.

Some functions of the brainstem

- The paramedian tegmental areas of the mesencephalon and rostral pons are deeply involved in arousal mechanisms ("generating the capacity for consciousness"). Strategically situated upper brainstem lesions cause permanent coma
- Respiratory drive
- Maintenance of blood pressure (spinal cord "centres" also involved) ⎤ → heart beat
- All motor outputs (cranial and somatic)
- All sensory inputs (except olfaction and vision)
- Sympathetic and parasympathetic efferents travel through the brainstem
- Cranial nerve reflexes readily testable

The irreversible cessation of respiration and heart beat implies death *of the patient as a whole*. It does not necessarily imply the immediate death *of every cell in the body*

The irreversible cessation of brainstem function implies death *of the brain as a whole.* It does not necessarily imply the immediate death *of every cell in the brain*

The difference between functional death (death of the organism as a whole) and total cellular death (death of the whole organism) has already been emphasised. The box summarises the parallel argument in relation to the brain as a whole and the whole brain.

Mechanisms of brainstem death

A severe head injury may be associated with cerebral oedema and a pronounced rise in intracranial pressure, even in the absence of a subdural or extradural haemorrhage. Similar rises (based on a different mechanism) may be seen after subarachnoid haemorrhage. Intracranial hypertension is also a feature of the cerebral oedema that almost invariably complicates acute anoxic insults to the brain. The initial effects, in such cases, are often complicated by the development of various intracranial "shifts." There may be downward spreading oedema and caudal displacement of the diencephalon and brainstem with stretching of the perforating pontine branches of the basilar artery and secondary haemorrhages in their territory, or the brainstem may be compressed from uncal herniation into the tentorial opening. Several factors may operate in any given case.

A pressure cone at the level of the foramen magnum may further damage the brainstem. Venous drainage may be compromised. Ischaemic changes may be striking. If ventilation is continued at room temperature in the presence of a dead brain, autolysis will occur. The whole brain may liquefy. Fragments of the destroyed cerebellar tonsils may become detached and be found even as far away as the roots of the cauda equina. The severity of the pathological changes may vary widely. Among the factors responsible for such variations are the duration of ventilation after arrest of the cerebral circulation and the proportion of cases, in some American series, which were not due to primary structural brain damage.

About half the patients in whom brainstem death is diagnosed in the United Kingdom have sustained a recent head injury. Another 30% have had a very recent intracranial haemorrhage (either intracerebral or subarachnoid).[27] Other primary intracranial conditions are meningitis or encephalitis. Not all such cases will be suitable as organ donors. In cases of cerebral tumour brainstem death may occur after operation or, rarely, when a prior decision has been taken, with the relatives'

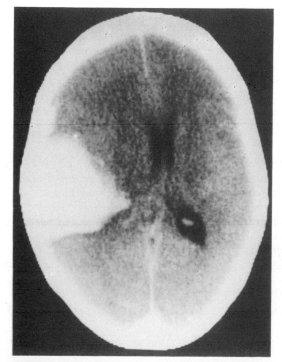
Computed tomogram of cerebral haematoma.

From brain death to brainstem death

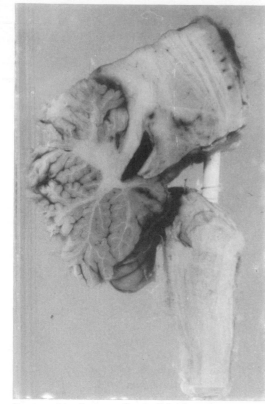

Ruptured brainstem after judicial hanging.

consent, to put the patient on a ventilator when in terminal coma (with the aim of making organs available for transplantation). Cardiac and respiratory arrest (and hypoperfusion of the brain complicating profound shock) are less common causes of brainstem death. They result more often in a persistent vegetative state.

Primary lesions of the brainstem (haemorrhages or infarcts) seldom cause total loss of brainstem function. Restricted lesions (causing restricted deficits) are more common. Massive lesions may occur, however, and result in brainstem death.

Judicial hanging is another cause of lethal, primary brainstem injury. Death in such cases is widely believed to be due to a fracture-dislocation of the odontoid with compression of the upper two segments of the spinal cord. Although such a lesion may be found in some cases, the late Professor Simpson, Home Office pathologist when capital punishment was still resorted to in the United Kingdom, informed one of us (CP) that a rupture of the brainstem (between pons and medulla) was more common.

In judicial hanging respiration stops immediately because of the effect of the rupture of the brainstem on the respiratory centre. Consciousness is also lost immediately as a result of the abrupt damage to the ascending reticular formation. The carotid or vertebral arteries may remain patent. The heart may go on beating for 20 minutes. Circulation continues, and parts of the brain are probably irrigated with blood (of diminishing oxygen saturation) for several minutes. We surmise that an electroencephalogram might, for a short while, continue to show some activity, despite the lethal injury to the brainstem. Is such a person alive or dead? The very posing of such a question forces one to focus attention on the reversibility or irreversibility of the inflicted brainstem lesion.

1 Horsley V. On the mode of death in cerebral compression and its prevention. *Quart Med J* 1894; July.
2 Duckworth D. Some cases of cerebral disease in which the function of respiration entirely ceases for some hours before that of the circulation. *Edinburgh Med J* 1898; 3:145–52.
3 Cushing H. Some experimental and clinical observations concerning states of increased intracranial tension. *Am J Med Sci* 1902; **124**:375–400.
4 Mollaret P, Goulon M. Le coma dépassé (mémoire préliminaire). *Rev Neurol (Paris)* 1959; **101**:3–15.
5 Wertheimer P, Jouvet M, Descotes J. A propos du diagnostic de la mort du système nerveux dans les comas avec arrêt respiratoire traités par la respiration artificielle. *Presse Med* 1959; **67**:87–8.
6 Ad Hoc Committee of the Harvard Medical School. A definition of irreversible coma. *JAMA* 1968; **205**:85–8.
7 Beecher HK. After the 'definition of irreversible coma'. *N Engl J Med* 1968; **281**:1070–1.
8 Mohandas A, Chou S N. Brain death — a clinical and pathological study. *J Neurosurg* 1971; **35**:211–8.
9 Babinski J. *Oeuvre scientifique* Paris:Masson, 1934:59.
10 Ivan LP. Spinal reflexes in cerebral death. *Neurology* 1973; **23**:650–2.
11 Jørgensen EO. Spinal man after brain death. *Acta Neurochir* (Wien) 1973; **28**:259–73.
12 Simpson K. The moment of death—a new medicolegal problem. *Acta Anaesthesiol Scand* 1968; **29** suppl:361–79.
13 Working Group of Conference of Medical Royal Colleges and their Faculties in the United Kingdom. Diagnosis of death. *BMJ* 1976; ii:1187–8.
14 Working Group of Conference of Medical Royal Colleges and their Faculties in the United Kingdom. Diagnosis of death. *BMJ* 1979; i:3320.
15 Working Group of Conference of Medical Royal Colleges and their Faculties in the United Kingdom. The criteria for the diagnosis of brainstem death. *J R Coll Phys (Lond)* 1995; **29**:381–2.
16 Byrne PA, O'Reilly S, Quay PM. Brain death — an opposing view. *JAMA* 1979; **242**:1985–90.
17 Evans DW, Lum LC. Cardiac transplantation. *Lancet* 1980; i:933–4.
18 Veith FJ, Fein JM, Tendler MD *et al.* Brain death. A status report of medical and ethical considerations. *JAMA* 1977; **238**:1651–5.
19 Smith AJK, Penry JK, eds. *Brain death: a bibliography with key-word and author indexes.* Bethesda: NINDS, 1972. (Bibliography series No 1.)
20 Korein J, ed. Brain death: interrelated medical and social issues. *Ann N Y Acad Sci* 1978; **315**:1–442.
21 Walker AE. *Cerebral death.* 2nd ed. Baltimore: Urban and Schwarzenberg, 1981.
22 Plum F. Organic disturbances of consciousness. In: Critchley M, Jennett B, eds. *Scientific foundations of neurology.* London:Heinemann, 1972.
23 Plum F, Posner JB. *The diagnosis of stupor and coma.* 3rd ed. Philadelphia: Davis, 1980.
24 Hass WK, Hawkins RA. Bilateral reticular formation lesions causing coma: their effects on regional blood-flow, glucose utilisation and oxidative metabolism. *Ann N Y Acad Sci* 1978; **315**:105–9.
25 Heiss WD, Jellinger K. Cerebral blow flow and brainstem lesion. *Zeitschrift Neurologie* 1972; **203**:197–209.
26 Ingvar DH, Sourander P. Destruction of the reticular core of the brainstem: a pathoanatomical follow-up of a case of coma of three years' duration. *Arch Neurol* 1970; **23**:1–8.
27 Jennett B, Hessett C. Brain death in Britain as reflected in renal donors. *BMJ* 1981; **283**:359–62.

3 DIAGNOSIS OF BRAINSTEM DEATH – 1

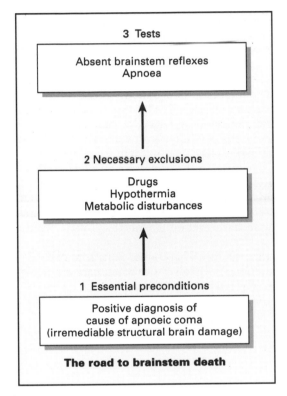

3 Tests

Absent brainstem reflexes
Apnoea

↑

2 Necessary exclusions

Drugs
Hypothermia
Metabolic disturbances

↑

1 Essential preconditions

Positive diagnosis of
cause of apnoeic coma
(irremediable structural brain damage)

The road to brainstem death

Three steps are involved in making a diagnosis of brainstem death:
- Ensuring that certain preconditions have been met
- Excluding reversible causes of apnoeic coma
- The clinical examination confirming brainstem areflexia and documenting persistent apnoea.

If every case is approached systematically errors should not occur. The aim of specifying preconditions and exclusions is much more subtle than is immediately apparent. They serve as a double filter. Once attention has been given to the preconditions and the exclusions, absence of brainstem function implies an irreversible state of affairs. "When near-misses are alleged, it usually transpires that the preconditions have not been stringently applied, rather than that tests had been inadequately performed."[1]

Preconditions

Two preconditions are necessary:
- That the patient is in apnoeic coma — that is, unresponsive and on a ventilator
- That the cause is irremediable structural brain damage due to a "disorder which can lead to brain death."

Several of these terms need elaboration.

Coma is a state of sleeplike unresponsiveness from which a patient cannot be roused. Such patients fail to open their eyes spontaneously, express no comprehensible words, and neither obey commands nor move their limbs appropriately to localise or resist painful stimulation (apnoeic coma, of course, precludes the possibility of testing phonation).[2 3] That the patient is on a ventilator should be self evident. The accurate determination of apnoea will be discussed later.

A positive diagnosis of a disorder that can lead to brain death depends on standard methods of history taking, clinical examination, and special investigation. Severe head injury and subarachnoid haemorrhage (which together account for about 80% of cases of brainstem death) are normally easy to diagnose. The patient is alert and well before rapidly becoming comatose. A history of cardiac arrest, strangulation, or drowning is not hard to establish either. If the primary diagnosis cannot be established the patient has not even approached the first hurdle: meeting the preconditions.

The objective is not only to diagnose a condition that could damage the brain but to establish that it has in fact done so irremediably. The *irremediable* nature of the damage is only partly assessed by the severity of the clinical features (apnoeic coma is always a critical state). In theory, irremediable means that no treatment may reasonably be expected to change the condition. In practice, it also means that no therapeutic endeavours (such as resuscitation or measures directed at

Preconditions

- Comatose patient on a ventilator

- Positive diagnosis of cause of coma (irremediable structural brain damage) controlling cerebral oedema) have changed the patient's condition during an adequate period of observation and that further endeavours are therefore unlikely to be effective. Detailed studies are now available relating eventual outcome to the failure of certain neurological signs to reappear during the critical first hour after cardiac arrest.[4][5] The passage of time is an essential component in determining that a lesion is irremediable; without it the term could easily become self serving.

Some remediable conditions may temporarily cause more severe neurological deficits than some irremediable ones. Subdural or extradural haematomas are potentially remediable. Massive intracerebral haemorrhage or gross destruction of the brain after trauma are not. Cerebral oedema may be remediable in its early stages but not after various mechanisms which reinforce its effects come into play.

The responsible disorder may be thought of as *structural* when it is not due to such functional — that is, potentially reversible — causes such as drug intoxication, hypothermia, or metabolic or endocrine disturbance. The structural nature of the disorder can usually be inferred from the history and clinical examination or established by direct inspection, imaging, or other investigations. Does establishing a diagnosis of structural brain disease necessarily imply visualizing a lesion or is inference of its structural nature enough? In a few cases cerebral oedema, reduction in ventricular size, or shifts due to brain swelling will have been shown by imaging or at surgery. Occasionally an open wound discloses the state of affairs. If the lesion is a subdural or extradural haematoma or an intracerebral haemorrhage there will, of course, be no problem.

Postanoxic oedema is another matter. The United Kingdom code rightly assumes that preconditions have been met when patients remain in coma and apnoeic for several hours after "successful" cardiopulmonary resuscitation. But trying to subsume the responsible lesions under the heading "structural" introduces unnecessary ambiguity. The American term "irreversible metabolic injury" would seem more appropriate.

> The passage of time is an essential component in determining that a lesion is **irremediable**

> The responsible lesion is deemed **structural** when no reversible causes are found, such as:
>
> - Drug intoxication
> - Hypothermia
> - Metabolic **or** endocrine disturbances

Exclusions

Drug intoxication, hypothermia, and metabolic or endocrine disturbances may all cause profound yet reversible changes in brainstem function. The United Kingdom code is unambiguous: brainstem death should *not* be considered in the presence of these conditions, whether they are primary causes of the coma or possible contributory factors in its perpetuation.

Acute intoxication is the commonest condition that needs to be excluded. Apart from head injury it is probably the commonest cause of a sudden coma lasting more than six hours in a previously healthy young adult. It is certainly the commonest cause of a deep coma of fairly rapid onset, still defying diagnosis 12 hours after admission to hospital. The initial history obtained from relatives is often unreliable. Most such patients will, of course, lack evidence of structural brain disease, even if in the deepest apnoeic coma. They will therefore not have crossed the "preconditions" hurdle. The diagnosis of brainstem death in patients maintained on a high barbiturate intake (as part of the "treatment" of their comatose state) cannot be established by purely clinical means. Resort to the testing of brainstem evoked potentials can be very useful in these circumstances (see chapter 8).

Problems may arise when the patient's state is suspected of being due to the combined effects of trauma and drugs. Common sense and clinical judgment are required. The circumstances are crucial. A depressed woman living alone and found unconscious at the foot of the stairs with a fractured skull is a different diagnostic problem from the healthy young climber who has slipped and sustained a similar fracture. A boxer knocked out in a ring and later lapsing into coma and a patient in hospital having a second subarachnoid bleed are easier to assess than the drunk who has fallen and knocked his head as he lurched out of a pub. Alcohol is the commonest (but only temporary) cause of diagnostic problems. The neurological effects of acute intoxication seldom last more than eight hours.

Physicians are still occasionally called to assess patients in intensive care units only to find that they are still under the influence of drugs

Coma and the duration of drug effects

Typical plasma half lives	(hours)
Phenobarbitone	100
Thiopentone	>24
Phenytoin	up to 140
Sodium valproate	7–10
Morphine	18–60
Fentanyl	2–4
Diamorphine	10–20
Ketamine	2–4
Tricyclic antidepressants	4–24
Carbamazepine	10–60
Diazepines	5–24
Phenothiazine derivatives	3–36
Antihistamines	6–24
Hypoglycaemic agents	2.5–36
Alcohol (fixed rate metabolism)	10 ml/hr

Always check with pharmacy information units
If in doubt, get plasma estimations done

blocking neuromuscular transmission. Efficient neuromuscular blockade will, of course, both produce apnoea and abolish most or all brainstem reflexes. The doctor called to the intensive care unit must always look at the drug sheet before testing for brainstem death.

If drug intoxication is suspected it is important to keep in mind the approximate plasma half lives of various drugs that produce coma and to remember that, as clearance proceeds, blood concentrations may fail to reflect brain concentrations. When toxicological facilities are not available — and there can be few major centres in the United Kingdom with facilities for ventilatory support but no access to a drug screening centre — it is reasonable to allow 48 to 72 hours for matters to sort themselves out. Unless the circumstances are absolutely clear cut there is no urgency about making a diagnosis of brainstem death. In practice trauma plus severe drug intoxication (other than alcohol) is rare.

A patient who has retained knee or ankle jerks cannot be under the influence of neuromuscular blocking drugs (the converse is not true). Very occasionally, because of rare inherited enzyme deficiencies the neuromuscular blockade may be prolonged. Doubts can be resolved (slowly) by allowing time to pass or (more promptly) by resort to a simple nerve stimulator. In patients with brainstem death there is no neuromuscular blockade. The peripheral nervous system is not affected and regular electrical stimuli applied to major nerve trunks will result in regular contractions of the muscles they supply.

The importance of timing

Timing

The time before testing

equals

The time taken

(a) to satisfy the preconditions
(b) to exclude drug intoxication, hypothermia, and severe metabolic disturbance

The United Kingdom code gives only general guidance on timing. This is as it should be. The "time before testing" (the time on the ventilator) is the time it takes to satisfy the preconditions and exclusions — that is, to establish an unequivocal diagnosis of structural brain damage and become certain that the condition is irremediable. An unhurried approach is the best safeguard against premature or unjustified suspicions of brainstem death.

Examples of observation periods in hours before testing ventilated patients

Apnoeic coma after	
● Major neurosurgery	
● Confirmed aneurysm. Second subarachnoid bleed in hospital	>4
Head injury (no secondary brain damage from haematoma, shock, or brain hypoxia)	>6
Spontaneous intracranial haemorrhage (without secondary hypoxic brain damage)	>6
Brain hypoxia (drowning, cardiac arrest, etc.)	>24
Any of the above (with suspicion of drug intoxication but no screening facilities)	50–100

The various clinical scenarios have been graphically described[1] but are worth recapitulating.

(1) When the patient develops persistent apnoeic coma in hospital — for example, after major neurosurgery or after a second bleed from an angiographically confirmed aneurysm — testing can be performed within a few hours.

(2) After a head injury immediate apnoea may develop. Most such patients die but occasionally artificial respiration is given at the scene of the accident. The patient may then recover spontaneous breathing after a few minutes. If apnoea develops after admission to the ward (secondary apnoea) the patient will usually be put on a ventilator while vigorous measures are taken to overcome the effects of hypoxia, shock, or cerebral oedema. Time must be allowed for these measures to take effect and for a raised blood alcohol concentration (if present) to subside below coma producing concentrations. It takes several hours to ensure that the responsible lesion is "irremediable." Testing for possible brainstem death in such cases is best deferred for at least six to 12 hours.

(3) Diagnosis of spontaneous intracranial haemorrhage (either subarachnoid or intracerebral) is usually straightforward, although accurate assessment may take several hours. Immediately after a first subarachnoid haemorrhage (or even occasionally after a second bleed) reversible apnoea may develop, lasting from a few minutes to an hour or so. When secondary apnoea develops after several hours in a case of intracranial haemorrhage the prognosis is grave as a pressure cone has probably developed. Both intracerebral and subarachnoid haemorrhage may lead to brainstem death, but it may take over six hours for the diagnosis of *irremediable*, structural brain damage to be unequivocally established.

(4) When a patient has suffered cerebral hypoxia after cardiac arrest or an anaesthetic accident the degree of brain damage may vary enormously. Even when the hypoxia has been severe (because of difficulties or delays in resuscitation) a vegetative state is a more common outcome than brainstem death. Persistent myoclonic seizures may develop within hours of the anoxic insult, and the effects of anticonvulsant drugs may then preclude reliable testing for irreversible loss of brainstem function. Recurrent episodes of hypotension or cerebral ischaemia may occur. Assessment may prove difficult and should not be hurried or take place too soon after the hypoxic insult. The United Kingdom code points out that "continuity of clinical observation and investigation" may be necessary before there is certainty that the preconditions have been fulfilled. This may take much longer than in cases of uncomplicated head injury, although there is now good evidence that the neurological prognosis after resuscitation from cardiac arrest (both in relation to brainstem death and to other forms of brain damage) may be ascertained earlier.[4][5]

(5) Longer periods of observation may occasionally be necessary when there is doubt about the possible contributory role of drugs (other than alcohol) or other confusing factors, such as hypothermia or metabolic upset. If the brainstem is dead many patients will develop asystole during this period. Cases in which the primary diagnosis is drug intoxication — that is, where there is no evidence of structural brain damage — will not, of course, have fulfilled the preconditions.

In each of these cases it is clearly up to the physician in charge to determine whether longer periods are necessary. The general philosophy prevailing in intensive care units should be that while the potential recipients of donated organs may be in a hurry, the donor never is.

1 Jennett B, Hessett C. Brain death in Britain as reflected in renal donors. *BMJ* 1981; **283**:359–62.
2 Plum F, Posner JB. *The diagnosis of stupor and coma.* 3rd ed. Philadelphia: Davis, 1980.
3 Levy DE, Bates D, Caronna JJ, *et al.* Prognosis in non-traumatic coma. *Ann Intern Med* 1981; **94**:293–301.
4 Jørgensen EO, Malchow-Møller A. Cerebral prognostic signs during cardiopulmonary resuscitation.. *Resuscitation* 1978; **6**:217–25.
5 Jørgensen EO, Malchow-Møller A. Natural history of global and critical brain ischaemia. II. EEG and neurological signs in patients remaining unconscious after resuscitation. *Resuscitation* 1981; **9**:155–74.

4   DIAGNOSIS OF BRAINSTEM DEATH – 2

The tests

Bedside tests

- Absent brainstem reflexes
- Apnoea (disconnection test)

Loss of brainstem function

Coma
No abnormal postures:
  - decorticate
  - decerebrate
No epileptic jerking
No brainstem reflexes
No spontaneous respiration

The tests necessary to show that the brainstem is not functioning take only a few minutes to carry out. They centre on proving that the brainstem reflexes have been lost and on scrupulous confirmation of persistent apnoea. If the preconditions for testing have been strictly adhered to and if reversible causes of brainstem dysfunction (such as hypothermia, drug intoxication, or metabolic disturbance) have been excluded the demonstration that the brainstem is not functioning is equivalent to asserting that the loss of function is irreversible — that the brainstem is dead.

As the physician approaches the bed he or she may notice signs which will immediately warn that the patient's brainstem cannot possibly be dead and that testing for brainstem death is therefore inappropriate. These signs will always be associated with retention of one or more of the brainstem reflexes, but detecting obviously relevant clues before formal testing is embarked on will prevent the physician wasting time.

A seizure, generalised or focal, implies the passage of nervous impulses through the brainstem and therefore proves that this part of the nervous system is still viable.

Abnormal postures, either "decorticate" (with flexed forearms and extended legs) or "decerebrate" (with extended and hyperpronated forearms and extended legs), likewise imply live neurones in the brainstem. Trismus has much the same importance.

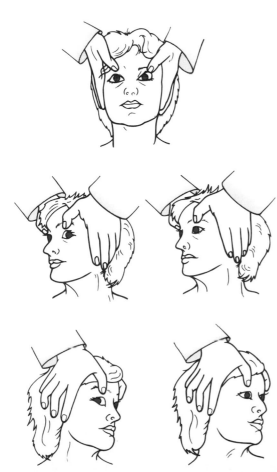

The presence of "dolling" (oculocephalic reflex or doll's head eye phenomenon) is important. Although this brainstem reflex is not mentioned in the United Kingdom code, an attempt to elicit it may save time. If there is a positive response the brainstem is alive, and there is no need to proceed with further testing. To elicit "dolling" the physician must get past the various wires, intravascular lines, and other impedimenta to the top of the bed and get between the wall and the patient's head. The physician then holds the patient's head between his or her hands and gently raises the lids with his or her thumbs. The head is then rotated first to one side (and kept there for three or four seconds while a close watch is kept on what happens to the eyes) and then through 180° right over in the opposite direction. (The test should not, of course, be done if there is any suspicion of cervical fracture as there will be in some patients after recent trauma.) In a fully alert person the eyes will, within a fraction of a second, orient with the head. In the cadaver the head and eyes will likewise move together. (In practice, there is no difficulty in distinguishing these two states.) If the patient has damaged cerebral hemispheres and a live brainstem the latter may show certain "release" phenomena. There will, for a second or two, be quite obvious deviation of the eyes to the opposite side as the head is rotated, followed by a prompt realignment of the eyes with the head. A similar dissociation will also occur when the head is then turned in the other direction. During each rotation the eyes are for a short while "out of phase" with the head. In the context of suspected brain death it is easier to perform the test properly if the patient is disconnected from the respirator for 20–30 seconds.

The brainstem reflexes

No brainstem reflexes

No pupillary response to light
No corneal reflex
No vestibulo-ocular reflex
No cranial nerve motor responses
No gag or reflex responses to tracheal
suction

(These five brainstem reflexes *must* be
absent before brainstem death can be
diagnosed)
Oculocephalic reflexes not specifically
mentioned in UK code. Test early for
"dolling" in every case. If present,
patient is clearly *not* brainstem dead

Five brainstem reflexes should then be tested systematically. There are certain basic requirements: a bright light for the pupillary responses; an adequate stimulus for the corneal reflexes; and a clear external auditory canal for caloric testing. The loss of response to stimulation as suction catheters are passed through the larynx and trachea will usually first have been detected by the nursing staff but should be confirmed in the presence of the examining physician.

The prescription that there should be "no motor response within the cranial nerve distribution" on "adequate stimulation of any somatic area" means, in practice, that there should be no grimacing in response to painful stimuli applied either to the trigeminal fields (firm supraorbital pressure) or to the limbs. Such grimacing implies that contact has been established in the brainstem between impulses coming in along various sensory pathways and cells in motor cranial nerve nuclei. Physicians are often unaware of how to apply painful stimuli to the limbs without leaving marks. The side of a pencil firmly pressed down against the patient's fingernail by the examiner's thumb is the ideal way. Pin pricks should never be used. A body covered with scratches is testimony of an examination carried out with more enthusiasm than skill.

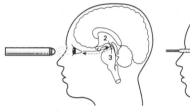 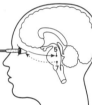 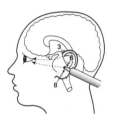

1 No pupillary response to light   2 No blinking on corneal touch   3 No eye movement on caloric testing

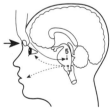 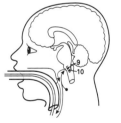

4 No grimacing on painful stimuli   5 No cough or gag reflex

Because the cranial nerve nuclei are so close to one another testing the brainstem reflexes enables the functional integrity of the brainstem to be probed in a unique way. No other area of the brain can be tested so thoroughly. This is fortunate because the concept of death proposed in chapter 1 implies that the two essential components of human life (the capacity for consciousness and the capacity to breathe) depend on the integrity of these few cubic centimetres of tissue.

Tests for brainstem reflexes fulfil the "criteria for good criteria" of death.[1] They yield vivid and unambiguous results. They look for the presence or absence of responses and not for gradations of function. They are simple to perform and capable of interpretation by any well trained doctor or nurse (and a fortiori by the highly trained physicians now required to carry them out). They do not depend on elaborate machinery, the vagaries of maintenance, or the presence around the clock of superspecialists. Their basis is easy to convey to both relatives and other lay people. Finally, they provide a battery of tests so that the determination of death does not rely exclusively on a single procedure or on the assessment of a single function.

Testing for apnoea

Problems in testing for apnoea

- Prevent hypoxia, which could further damage the brain
- Ensure that the Pa_{CO_2} builds up to critical level

The ultimate test of brainstem function is the test for apnoea. Apnoea is established by showing that no respiratory movements occur during disconnection from the ventilator for long enough to ensure that the arterial carbon dioxide tension (Pa_{CO_2}) rises to a level capable of driving any respiratory centre neurones that may still be alive. Two main problems will immediately be apparent: how to prevent hypoxia which could of itself damage the brain; and how to ensure that the Pa_{CO_2} does in fact build up to the critical level during the period of disconnection.

Hypoxia can be prevented if the patient is preoxygenated with 100% oxygen for 10 minutes before testing and diffusion oxygenation is then maintained throughout the disconnection procedure. Provided that there is no gross diffusion defect in the lungs, breathing 100% oxygen for 10 minutes will wash out the body nitrogen, saturate the tissues with oxygen, and build up a high arterial oxygen partial pressure

Testing for apnoea

- Preoxygenate with 100% oxygen for 10 minutes
- Reduce ventilation rate or administer 5% CO_2 with 95% oxygen if Pa_{CO_2} before test is less than 5.3 kPa (40 mm Hg)
- Disconnect, insufflate with 100% oxygen at 6 l/min through intratracheal catheter passed to carina
- Maintain disconnection for a period sufficient to ensure that the Pa_{CO_2} reaches 6.5 kPa (50 mm Hg)

(Pa_{O_2}), which will remain adequate during the period of apnoea. Diffusion oxygenation is ensured by delivering oxygen (at 6 l/min) by a catheter down the trachea. The physiological basis of these procedures was established many years ago[2-4] and has been repeatedly confirmed.

To ensure that the Pa_{CO_2} reaches levels adequate to stimulate the respiratory centre during the period off the ventilator the patient must not be hypocapnic at the time of disconnection. Patients in intensive care units tend to be overventilated. They may run continuous Pa_{CO_2} levels well below 4 kPa (30 mm Hg). There are two ways of overcoming this hypocapnoea: by slowing the rate of the ventilator or ventilating the patient with 5% carbon dioxide in 95% oxygen for five minutes before disconnection. This will raise the Pa_{CO_2} to at least 5.3 kPa (40 mm Hg).

During the period of disconnection the Pa_{CO_2} will increase still further. The rise is slow in immobile, moderately hypothermic patients who often have depressed metabolic rates but is at least 0.27 kPa (2 mm Hg) per minute. Most authors in fact report that the rate of increase is faster than this.[5-7] Ten minutes' disconnection will raise the Pa_{CO_2} by at least another 2.7 kPa (20 mm Hg). A Pa_{CO_2} of 8.0 kPa (60 mm Hg) will then have been reached, which is more than enough to drive a respiratory centre capable of responding to a hypercarbic stimulus. The Pa_{CO_2} achieved (at the end of the period of disconnection) should be recorded.

The United Kingdom code recommends that during disconnection the Pa_{CO_2} should rise to at least 6.65 kPa (50 mm Hg) before the patient is deemed incapable of breathing. A recent study has re-emphasised that this is an adequate level.[7] The continuous administration of 5% carbon dioxide for a few minutes before disconnection will in fact ensure that the Pa_{CO_2} at the end of disconnection will have risen to at least 8.0 kPa (60 mm Hg). This administration of 5% carbon dioxide is strongly recommended when there are no facilities for blood gas analysis.

The test for apnoea may be the most critical of all tests of brainstem function. Testing for apnoea without ensuring and documenting an appropriate rise in Pa_{CO_2} has been likened to "testing the pupils without a battery in the torch."[8] Some patients in coma due to structural brain damage may have lost all their brainstem reflexes yet may (for a short while) retain their capacity to take a few spontaneous breaths when suitably stimulated.[6] So long as this capacity persists the brainstem cannot be said to be dead. This should lead one to question some of the conclusions drawn from studies which were not scrupulous (or constant) in their definition of apnoea — for instance, work defining apnoea as the patient making "no effort to override the respirator"[9] or leaving the duration of disconnection "to the judgment of the attending physician."[10] It is even harder to assess work seriously which states that the operational concept of apnoea (in patients being tested to ascertain brain death) "does not in any way imply absent respiratory centre function."[10]

There remain a few patients suffering from chronic obstructive airway disease who may be dependent on an anoxic drive to respiration. It is difficult to assess the function of their respiratory centre properly. The United Kingdom code describes them as special cases who "should be expertly investigated with careful blood gas monitoring." When possible this should clearly be done, but it is probably a counsel of perfection for on many occasions such facilities will not exist. It would require frequent and rapid, if not continuous, monitoring of Pa_{O_2}, with monitoring also of mixed venous samples via a pulmonary catheter. The danger is more hypoxic damage to the brain and to those organs being considered for donation. There is also the difficulty of knowing what level of hypoxia for a given patient represents an adequate stimulus. One would logically and ideally need to know the patient's Pa_{O_2} before admission to hospital. This is rarely available except in those patients who have been admitted to or attended the hospital on a regular basis. The usual Pa_{O_2} figure quoted as being the "danger level" for cerebral damage is 5.3 kPa. Most such patients will probably not be considered for a diagnosis of brainstem death.

Repetition of testing

Virtually all codes urge that testing be carried out twice. The recommended intervals between the relevant tests have progressively shortened. There are several reasons why this has happened. Firstly, the objections to ventilating corpses have become more widely accepted. Secondly, when the first and second examinations for brain death were separated by as long as 24 hours several patients would develop asystole before the second examination. Finally, it became widely recognised that provided scrupulous attention was given to the preconditions and exclusions the second examination always confirmed the first. In other words, the more time spent before the first testing in ascertaining the irremediable nature of the structural brain damage causing the coma the less important does the interval between tests become.

What is the purpose of retesting in a patient with a non-functioning brainstem due to well established, irremediable, structural brain damage? The United Kingdom code claims that it is to ensure that there has been no observer error. This is entirely praiseworthy, although no properly documented case has been published where the diagnosis of brainstem death has been revised after repeat testing. In our opinion retesting usually has a different purpose. It ensures that the non-functioning of the brainstem is not just a single observation at one point in time but that it has persisted. For how long? For a period several hundredfold that during which brainstem neurones could survive the total ischaemia of a non-perfused brain. At Hammersmith Hospital we like to separate our tests by two to three hours, which is more than enough to ensure that the findings are irreversible.

Purposes of retesting

No observer error
No change in signs

---

1 Task Force on Death and Dying of the Institute of Society, Ethics, and Life Sciences. Refinements in criteria for the determination of death: an appraisal. *JAMA* 1972; **221**:48–53.
2 Enghoff H, Holmdahl MH, Risholm M. Diffusion respiration in man. *Nature* 1951; **168**:830.
3 Frumin MJ, Epstein RM, Cohen G. Apnoeic oxygenation in man. *Anaesthesiology* 1959; **20**:789–98.
4 Payne JP. Apnoeic oxygenation in anaesthetised man. *Acta Anaesthiol Scand* 1962; **6**:129–42.
5 Milhaud A, Riboulot M, Gayet H. Disconnecting tests and oxygen uptake in the diagnosis of total brain death. *Ann N Y Acad Sci* 1978; **315**:241–51.
6 Schafer JA, Caronna JJ. Duration of apnoea needed to confirm brain death. *Neurology* 1978; **28**:661-6.
7 Ropper AH, Kennedy SK, Russell L. Apnoea testing in the diagnosis of brain death. Clinical and physiological observations. *J Neurosurg* 1981; **55**:942–6.
8 Whitwam JG. Brain death. *Lancet* 1980; **ii**:1142.
9 Anonymous. An appraisal of the criteria of cerebral death. *JAMA* 1977; **237**:982–6.
10 Bennett DR, Hughes, JR, Korein J, *et al. Atlas of electroencephalography in coma and cerebral death.* New York: Raven Press, 1976.

5 PITFALLS AND SAFEGUARDS

Pitfalls in diagnosis

> **Pitfalls in diagnosis**
>
> - Meeting preconditions and exclusions
> - Technique of eliciting signs
> - Interpretation of signs elicited

Criteria of brainstem death can be judged fairly only when they are correctly applied. The basic truth that we all make mistakes should not be allowed to blur the difference between fallible physicians and fallacious criteria. Past controversies have, if anything, re-emphasised the soundness of criteria used in the United Kingdom code. The adoption of similar criteria in other countries points in the same direction. Nevertheless, it is necessary to be aware of potential pitfalls. These fall into three broad categories: failure to ensure that preconditions and exclusions have been met; technical errors in testing; and mistakes in interpreting observed signs.

Failure to fulfil the preconditions

> **Failure to fulfil the preconditions**
>
> Is there:
> - A comatose patient on a ventilator?
> - An unequivocally established cause for the coma?
> - Irremediable, structural brain damage?

Failure to fulfil the preconditions is the commonest pitfall. To recommend that "it is almost [sic] always desirable to have an aetiologic basis for the diagnosis"[1] is asking for trouble. Testing for brainstem death should not be undertaken unless the cause of the coma has been established beyond all doubt. The United Kingdom code restricts the range of acceptable causes (by specifying which conditions should be excluded). It also emphasises the importance of timing.

Eliciting and interpreting signs

> **Eliciting and interpreting signs**
>
> - Is the stimulus adequate?
> - Have anticholinergic drugs been given?
> - Have mydriatics been used?
> - Could the unreactive pupil be due to pre-existing disease?
> - Has the patient a glass eye?

The pupils

Despite the requirements of several earlier codes it is not necessary for the pupils to be dilated. Mydriasis is not a feature of a dead brain, as can readily be ascertained in any morgue.[2] When the brainstem is dead the pupils are usually in the mid-position. The important point is that they should show no response to light. A really bright light is needed: household torches or ophthalmoscopes should not be used as sources of light. It is also advisable to darken the room.

Widely dilated, unresponsive pupils may be caused by atropine administered in the course of cardiac resuscitation. The effects may persist for several hours. Errors may also arise when topical mydriatics are instilled (to facilitate examination of the fundi) and the fact not recorded in the notes. Pre-existing ocular or neurological disease may account for the pupils failing to respond to light, as may local damage to the globe or nerves to the eye due to craniofacial injury.

Corneal reflexes

Testing corneal reflexes in patients with suspected brainstem death requires much firmer pressure than is used in conscious patients. Delicate dabbing with a wisp of cotton wool does not really provide adequate stimulus. A sterile throat swab is more suitable. Overenthusiastic testing, however, may damage the corneas and render them unsuitable for donation.

Pitfalls and safeguards

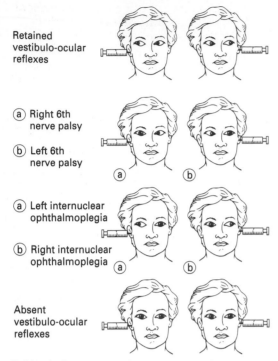

Retained vestibulo-ocular reflexes

(a) Right 6th nerve palsy

(b) Left 6th nerve palsy

(a) Left internuclear ophthalmoplegia

(b) Right internuclear ophthalmoplegia

Absent vestibulo-ocular reflexes

Cold caloric responses in comatose patients.

Apnoea on disconnection

- Post-hyperventilation apnoea?
- Persistent neuromuscular blockade?

Some pitfalls in the diagnosis of brain death

Finding	Possible cause
Pupils fixed	Anticholinergic drugs Neuromuscular blockers Pre-existing disease
No vestibulo-ocular (caloric) reflexes	Ototoxic agents Vestibular suppressants Pre-existing disease Skull fracture through petrous temporal bone
No respiration	Apnoea after hyperventilation Neuromuscular blockers
No motor activity	Neuromuscular blockers "Locked in" state Sedative drugs
Isoelectric electro-encephalogram	Sedative drugs Anoxia Hypothermia Encephalitis Trauma

---

Caloric testing

Caloric testing requires a wax-free external auditory canal, verified with an otoscope at the time of testing. The United Kingdom code recommends irrigation of the tympanic membrane with 20 ml of ice cold water. More may be used if the examiner thinks the whole volume has not been directed at the tympanum. If there is a large perforation — and the patient still has a functioning brainstem — a fall in blood pressure and bradycardia may occur. The stimulus should elicit no movement whatsoever in either eye. Tonic deviation towards the irrigated side, even if confined to one eye, implies that part of the brainstem is still alive. (Deviation confined to the ipsilateral eye indicates a contralateral internuclear ophthalmoplegia, and deviation confined to the contralateral eye suggests a sixth nerve palsy on the stimulated side). In unconscious patients there is unlikely to be any fast "corrective" jerking away from the side of the irrigated ear. Occasionally, failure to elicit ocular movement in response to irrigation of the tympanic membranes with iced water is due to end organ poisoning — for instance, from antibiotics such as gentamicin — or to end organ disease. The central mechanisms responsible for the vestibulo-ocular reflexes may be impaired or suppressed by drugs, including sedatives, anticholinergics, anticonvulsants, and tricyclic antidepressants.

Apnoea

The technical aspects of testing have already been described. Interpreting the results may occasionally cause difficulties. Excessive ventilation (resulting in a low Pa_{CO_2}) is a potentially confusing cause of reluctance to breathe. Apnoea after hyperventilation is unlikely to cause diagnostic problems if the blood gases are measured before disconnection. At the time of disconnection the Pa_{CO_2} should be at least 5.3 kPa (40 mm Hg). If there are no facilities for determination of blood gases the patient should (as previously described) be ventilated with 5% carbon dioxide in oxygen for a few minutes before disconnection to ensure an appropriate "starting" level. Patients with chronic obstructive airways disease may depend in whole or in part on a hypoxic stimulus to respiration and may fail to breathe at what would otherwise be appropriate levels of Pa_{CO_2}. Great care is necessary in determining brainstem death in such cases, but patients with major respiratory problems sufficient to make testing difficult will probably not be suitable for solid organ donation (see also chapter 4). Severe problems may occur with intrapulmonary shunting in patients with major chest injuries in whom adequate oxygenation is not possible. Unacceptable hypoxia may occur during testing. As in every case when there is doubt about the validity of any part of the brainstem testing the tests should be abandoned. Prolonged apnoea may very occasionally occur when neuromuscular blocking agents are given to patients lacking the appropriate inactivating enzymes. The drugs will usually have been given to assist intubation or the management of emergency obstruction. The use of the nerve stimulator to recognise this state of affairs has already been mentioned.

Motor function

Motor function may be impaired in the limbs (and the tendon reflexes reduced or abolished) as a result of neuromuscular blocking drugs or of large doses of sedatives. Either or both may have been prescribed by anaesthetists "to prevent the patient from struggling against the ventilator" (the very use of such terms suggests that the patient's brainstem is alive). Inquiries should always be made as to when the last dose of such drugs was given.

In practice these pitfalls are easy to avoid, and genuine diagnostic problems are rare. They arise only when several factors contribute to the overall clinical condition — for example, when patients with severe polyneuritis sustain anoxic insults from ventilatory accidents or when patients in drug induced coma suffer cardiac arrest. Most other problems are of the hypothetical type beloved of ingenious students but which nature seldom produces. The number of cases of subarachnoid haemorrhage occurring in tabetic patients with chronic bronchitis intoxicated with gentamicin must be very small.

Three conditions will be mentioned, not because of any profound clinical resemblance to brainstem death but because they are repeatedly brought up in theoretical discussions of the subject.

Brainstem encephalitis may result in severe external (and sometimes internal) ophthalmoplegia, facial diplegia, and bulbar palsy.[3-5] The patients may be drowsy but are not in deep coma. Several brainstem reflexes may be absent. But there is no significant motor or sensory deficit in the arms or legs, which are moved spontaneously or briskly withdrawn on stimulation. Ataxia is pronounced. Breathing is occasionally affected. The overall clinical picture is striking: "an apparently moribund patient who can use his limbs to operate suction apparatus to remove secretions accumulated in his throat."[3]

Idiopathic polyneuritis (Guillain-Barré syndrome) — In this condition cranial nerve involvement and respiratory paralysis are well recognised, although ophthalmoplegia is rare.[6-8] The history will again be characteristic, motor and sensory symptoms in the limbs usually being prominent.

Ventral pontine infarction may lead to the "locked in syndrome." Bilateral lesions of the corticospinal and corticobulbar pathways render the patient tetraplegic and aphonic. There will be bilateral pyramidal signs. Consciousness and alertness are retained as are conjugate vertical gaze and (usually) the capacity to blink. Hearing is unaffected. The patients perceive pain normally and breathe spontaneously.

As repeatedly emphasised, the history and context are paramount in diagnosing brainstem death. Only when they are ignored and signs of brainstem dysfunction are assessed in isolation rather than in context can confusion conceivably arise. If the diagnosis of brainstem death is envisaged only in cases of known head injury, cerebrovascular accidents, or hypoxic encephalopathy there should be no diagnostic errors.

Other conditions

- Brainstem encephalitis
- Guillain-Barré syndrome
- Ventral pontine infarction ("locked in" state)

Paediatric problems

Diagnosis of brainstem death in neonates and small babies is fraught with difficulties. In 1988 a working party of the Conference of Medical Royal Colleges addressed the issue of "Organ Transplantation in Neonates." Their report concluded that "in view of the current uncertainties, organs for transplantation should not be removed within the first seven days of life from neonates with beating hearts, even if they satisfy the brainstem death criteria which are used in older children and adults."[9]

Three years later the matter was taken further in a working party report of the British Paediatric Association. Of infants less than 2 months old the report had concluded that "given the current state of knowledge it is rarely possible confidently to diagnose brainstem death at this age."[10] Below 37 weeks' gestation they thought that "the concept of brainstem death was inappropriate." Discussing electrophysiological measurements in infants and children the working party "did not feel confident, given the current state of knowledge, that the investigations were a helpful addition to the diagnosis of brainstem death."

An American view, summarised by Ashwal and Schneider in a series of articles,[11-13] described criteria identical with those for the establishment of brain death in adults.

There is still some disagreement concerning the ability of the newborn to withstand prolonged hypoxic insults. There may be a greater capacity for the immature brain to withstand anoxia, and the unfused skull of the infant can certainly accommodate a swollen brain more easily. Once the clinical features of a dead brainstem are present, however, it is doubtful whether the cardiac prognosis is any different.

Premature neurological or electrophysiological assessments after anoxic insult may be particularly misleading in children. A case is on record of a child aged 28 months who became severely hypoxic after dislocation of a tracheostomy cannula inserted for bronchopulmonary dysplasia. On reaching an intensive care unit the child was incapable of

---

Criteria for the determination of brain death in children

- Do not diagnose under 7 days (care needed under 5 years)
- Identified cause of the coma
- Exclude toxic and metabolic causes
- Core temperature at least 36.1°C
- Normotensive, normovolemic
- Absent brainstem reflexes
- Apnoea with $Paco_2$ rising to 60 mm Hg or more

breathing spontaneously. Initially fixed and dilated pupils were now reacting. An electroencephalogram (two hours after resuscitation) was said to have shown "electrocerebral silence." There was also loss of brainstem auditory evoked potential waves IV and V. The electroencephalogram and brainstem auditory evoked potentials became normal during the next 18 hours. After 35 hours complete brainstem areflexia developed, the apnoea test was positive, and the child disconnected from the ventilator.[14] This illustrates a point in the United Kingdom code which specifies that when suspected brainstem death occurs in the context of "an indefinite period of cerebral anoxia" it may take more than a few hours to "establish the diagnosis and be confident of the prognosis."

In the United States the task force for the determination of brain death in children emphasised that the newborn were clinically difficult to assess after perinatal insults.[15] There was often difficulty in determining the proximate cause of the coma, and the validity of laboratory tests was uncertain. The President's Commission warned physicians to be "particularly cautious in applying neurological criteria to determine death in children aged younger than 5 years."[16] Even after advances made since then the warning remains valid.

The use of organs from anencephalic infants has been considered in Britain by the Conference of Medical Royal Colleges, who recommended that organs from such infants may be used when two doctors who are not members of the transplant team agree that spontaneous respiration has ceased.[9] This is not a universally held view. In Holland the use of tissues or organs from foetus or anencephalic infants is not permitted (I R de Jong, personal communication). A meeting in Canada to discuss the topic agreed that the absence of spontaneous respiration would signify death but warned that use of organs from anencephalic infants might face the same legal and ethical problems we find with other donors.[17] In the United States the experience has been that parents are only too willing to consider an anencephalic infant as an organ donor. Nevertheless, there seem to be no guidelines there on any legal issues concerned, although it has been pointed out that there is a moral imperative that treatment of the infant as a patient takes precedence over the need for organs, however acute that need. In a review of the problem the United Network for Organ Sharing (UNOS), which administers the network in the United States, considered that "the anencephalic is not an exception to the usual criteria and procedures for organ donation" and "anencephaly should not be considered a state that in and of itself warrants organ donation."[18] That seems a reasonable summary.

Safeguards for the patient

If there is any doubt about:

- the primary diagnosis
- the possible contribution of reversible factors, hypothermia, drugs, metabolic disorders

then

DO NOT DIAGNOSE BRAINSTEM DEATH

Conclusion

To diagnose as still alive someone who is already dead must sometimes be accepted, for a while. Reality will soon reassert itself. Such an error is the price we pay for avoiding the opposite error. There must always be the most stringent safeguards for the patient, and the benefit of any doubt must always be exercised in his or her favour.

No diagnosis of brainstem death should, in our view, be made if the physician in charge of the case still has any doubts about:

- the primary diagnosis
- the possible contributory role of reversible causes of brainstem dysfunction (such as hypothermia, drugs, or metabolic upset)
- the adequacy or completeness of the clinical testing.

There will be general agreement about the first two points but argument may arise on the third. The patient may have a fractured skull and cerebrospinal fluid otorrhoea, precluding caloric testing. Or there may be extensive facial injuries rendering difficult the proper testing of the pupillary or corneal reflexes. More prosaically the patient may have a glass eye. All or any of these may restrict the number of cranial nerves that can be tested. Is it permissible to diagnose irreversible loss of brainstem function on clinical grounds on the basis of partial data? Some would argue that it is not. Others would point out that provided there is no doubt about the preconditions and exclusions and provided apnoea has been rigorously confirmed there is sufficient redundancy in the tests to allow the diagnosis to be made. They would also emphasise that guidelines are no more than what they claim to be, that they are not edicts to be followed to the letter, that in a given context the answer is usually quite simple, and that all data — whether complete or not — should be interpreted, as in other specialties of medicine, with common sense by experienced and humane physicians.

1 Korein J. The problem of brain death: development and history. *Ann N Y Acad Sci* 1978; **315**:19–38.
2 Plum F, Posner JB. *The diagnosis of stupor and coma*. 3rd ed. Philadelphia: Davis, 1980.
3 Al-Din AN, Anderson M, Bickerstaff ER, Harvey I. Brainstem encephalitis and the syndrome of Miller-Fisher. *Brain* 1982; **105**:481–95.
4 Chandler JM, Brilli RJ. Brainstem encephalitis imitating brain death. *Crit Care Med* 1991; **19**:977–9.
5 Ragosta K. Miller-Fisher syndrome, a brainstem encephalitis, mimics brain death. *Clin Pediatr (Phila)* 1993; **32**:685–7.
6 Marti-Masso JF, *et al*. Clinical signs of brain death simulated by Guillain-Barré syndrome. *J Neurol Sci* 1993; **120**:115–7.
7 Coad NR, Bryne AJ, Guillain-Barré syndrome mimicking brainstem death. *Anaesthesia* 1990; **45**:456–7.
8 Hassan T, Mumford C. Guillain-Barré syndrome mistaken for brainstem death. *Postgrad Med J* 1991; **67**:280–1.
9 Working Party on Organ Transplantation in Neonates. *Report of Conference of medical Royal Colleges and their faculties in the UK*. London: Department of Health and Social Security, 1988.
10 Working Party of the British Paediatric Association. *Diagnosis of brainstem death in infants and children*. London: British Paediatric Association, 1991.
11 Ashwal S, Schneider S. Brain death in children. *Pediatr Neurol* 1987 **3**:5–11.
12 Ashwal S, Schneider S. Brain death in children. *Pediatr Neurol* 1987 **3**:69–77.
13 Ashwal S, Schneider S. Brain death in the new born. *Pediatrics* 1989 **84**:429–37.
14 Schmitt B, Simma B, Burger R, Dummermuth G. Resuscitation after severe hypoxia in a young child: temporary isoelectric EEG and loss of BAEP components. *Intensive Care Med* 1993; **19**:420–2.
15 Task Force for the Determination of Brain Death in Children. Guidelines for the determination of brain death in children. *Arch Neurol* 1987; **44**:587–8.
16 Medical Consultants on the diagnosis of death to the President's Commission for the Study of Ethical Problems in Medicine and Behavioral Research. Guidelines for the determination of death. *JAMA* 1981; **246**:2185–6.
17 Stiller CR. International consensus on anencephalic donors. *Transplant Proc* 1988; **20** (suppl 5) 1–83.
18 Ethics Committee. *The anencephalic infant as an organ source: medical and ethical considerations*. Virginia, United States: United Network for Organ Sharing, 1989.

6 THE DECLARATION OF DEATH

Unnecessary anguish and distress to relatives and nurses may be caused by insensitive or thoughtless handling of brain dead patients. Inadequate or conflicting statements (or a failure to explain anything whatsoever about what is happening) often prove to be the basis for sensationalisation of the issue by the media and for a great deal of ill informed talk about "pulling the plug out," "discontinuing life support," and so on. A correct approach should make it abundantly clear (both to relatives and to a wider public) that in the act of disconnection "the doctor is not withdrawing treatment and allowing someone to die, but ceasing to do something useless to someone who is already dead."[1]

If a comatose patient on a ventilator is thought to have reached the stage of brainstem death the doctor in charge of the case should seek to confirm the diagnosis using accepted criteria. The United Kingdom code recommends that the tests should be carried out by two medical practitioners who have skill in this field. One should be a consultant and the other a consultant or senior registrar.[2]

In practice these doctors will often be anaesthetists, neurologists, neurosurgeons, or intensive care physicians, but this is certainly not essential. Any physician of appropriate seniority who has understood the preconditions can perform the tests. A survey showed that in the United Kingdom 45% of brain dead kidney donors came from non-teaching hospitals without neurosurgical facilities. It is our view that by the end of the millennium every medical student should be able to recognise when a comatose patient has a dead brainstem. The idea that neurologists or other specialists should carry out the necessary confirmatory tests will then seem as bizarre as would the notion today that two cardiologists are needed to diagnose death on conventional grounds.

As soon as they have completed their first examination the doctors concerned should write down their findings in the patient's notes or on the special checklists that are available. The time of the testing should be carefully recorded, as should the nature of the irremediable structural brain damage and the duration of apnoeic coma. The entry should then describe, serially, the results of testing the brainstem reflexes. It should confirm that a disconnection test for apnoea was performed. If the Pa_{CO_2} was estimated at the end of the disconnection period, as is advisable, the result should be recorded. It is sound and helpful to perform the disconnection test as the last of the tests of brainstem function. Sometimes — provided there has been no tendency whatsoever to reflex movements of spinal origin and the patient has

---

CHECKLIST OF CRITERIA FOR DIAGNOSIS OF BRAINSTEM DEATH

Diagnosis to be made by two independent doctors one a consultant and the other a consultant or senior registrar. Diagnosis should not normally be considered until at least 6 hours after the onset of coma or, if cardiac arrest was the cause of the coma, until 24 hours after the circulation has been restored.

Name ....   Unit No ....

PRE-CONDITIONS

Are you satisfied that the patient suffers from a condition that has led to irremediable brain damage? Specify the condition :	Time of onset of unresponsive coma :
Dr A	....
Dr B	....

Are you satisfied that potentially reversible causes for the patient's condition have been adequately excluded, in particular :

	Dr A	Dr B
Depressant drugs		
Neuromuscular blocking (relaxant) drugs		
Hypothermia		
Metabolic or endocrine disturbances		

TESTS FOR ABSENCE OF BRAIN-STEM FUNCTION

	Dr A 1st testing	Dr A 2nd testing	Dr B 1st testing	Dr B 2nd testing
Do the pupils react to light?				
Are there corneal reflexes?				
Is there eye movement on caloric testing?				
Are there motor responses in the cranial nerve distribution, in response to stimulation of face, limbs or trunk?				
Is there a gag reflex? (If the test is practicable)				
Is there a cough reflex?				
Have the recommendations concerning testing for apnoea been followed?*				
Were any respiratory movements seen?				

	Dr A	Dr B
Date and time of first testing		
Date and time of second testing		

(As stated in paragraph 30 of the Code of Practice the two doctors may carry out the tests separately or together.)

Dr A Signature ....   Dr B Signature ....

Status ....   Status ....

*Diagnosis of Brain Death. Brit Med J 1976, ii, 1187-8.
See note (b) on page 35 of the Code of Practice

been adequately pre-oxygenated — it is useful for the relatives to witness the first disconnection test. It helps them understand the difference between breathing and "being breathed." It also helps them perceive the implications of the condition and accept that a declaration of death is probably imminent.

After the first clinical testing the patient will have been reconnected to the ventilator. A second testing should be carried out, the interval between the tests being left to the judgment of the doctors concerned (see chapter 4). If the second testing confirms a dead brainstem, death should be declared, the relatives notified, and a further appropriate entry made in the notes. A patient is dead when a doctor (using accepted criteria) declares him or her to be dead. Legally, this is deemed to be the time of death. A death certificate should then be issued. This is a good way of making it clear that any continued ventilation, administration of fluids, or drug treatment is not aimed at treating the patient (who is dead) but at optimising the condition of organs likely to be used for transplantation.

If organ donation is not envisaged there is no need to reconnect the cadaver to the ventilator. The second test apnoea will have merged with permanent disconnection. If transplantation is planned the "beating heart cadaver" should be reconnected to the ventilator. The organ retrieval can then be carried out at the convenience of the surgical team. Only exceptionally should artificial ventilation have to be maintained for more than a few hours after a declaration of brainstem death. The main consideration is to ensure that the potential recipients receive organs in as good a condition as possible. The detailed management of the potential donor is covered in chapter 10.

To minimise the risk of possible later misunderstandings all disconnections are best performed by doctors not nurses. There are no reasons in logic for this recommendation, but the whole subject is one in which irrational behaviour is still occasionally encountered.

Declaration of brainstem death

- Have the preconditions been met?
- Is the patient comatose and on a ventilator?
- Is there a positive diagnosis of irremediable structural brain damage?
- Have the necessary exclusions been rigorously observed?
- Has each of two examinations shown:
  Absent brainstem reflexes?
  Persistent apnoea on disconnection?
- If so, the patient can be declared dead; once the patient has been declared dead, the patient is effectively a ventilated cadaver
- The patient is dead when the brainstem is declared dead and not when ventilation is stopped and the heart stops beating
- Electroencephalography, angiography, or other tests of brain "perfusion" are not required for a diagnosis of brainstem death

1 Jennett B, Hessett C. Brain death in Britain as reflected in renal donors. *BMJ* 1981; **283**:359–62.
2 Robson JG. Brain death. *Lancet* 1981; **ii**:364.

7 PROGNOSTIC SIGNIFICANCE OF A DEAD BRAINSTEM

In 1983, in the first edition of this book, a concept of human death was proposed as "the irreversible loss of the capacity for consciousness combined with the irreversible loss of the capacity to breathe." This concept has now been officially endorsed.[1] That a permanently non-functioning brainstem could provide the necessary and sufficient substratum for such a state is a matter of anatomy and physiology. It might seem strange at first sight now to start discussing the prognosis of a corpse.

There is, however, merit in discovering whether brainstem death invariably heralds asystole and how soon. Firstly, to establish a link between the past and present concepts of death; secondly, to reassure those who still believe that "real" or "ultimate" death occurs only when the circulation ceases and who would prefer a foot in both camps; and, finally, to answer critics' claims that we do not know the cardiac prognosis of those with dead brainstems and even that diagnosing the condition leads to disconnecting patients and that a "fatal" outcome in the brain dead is therefore a self fulfilling prophecy.

Ventilating to asystole

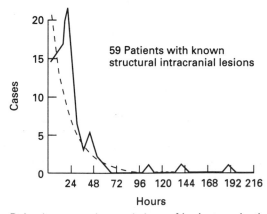

59 Patients with known structural intracranial lesions

Delay between observed signs of brainstem death and development of isoelectric electroencephalogram.

Papers written in the late 1960s leave no doubt that many patients fulfilling criteria of the Harvard type were still being ventilated for hours or days. Every neurological, neurosurgical, and intensive care unit did not immediately and without question accept the new criteria of death and start "switching off" all patients who met them. Questionnaires sent out in 1969 by the American Electroencephalography Society to its own members (and to many neurologists) disclosed that at least 15% of the 405 neurologists who responded "insisted on traditional cardiorespiratory cessation for declaration of death."[2] These physicians were presumably ventilating their comatose and apnoeic patients until the heart stopped. In the tense and controversy ridden years that followed the Harvard report news of any "recoveries" would undoubtedly have leaked out and been seized on by the media, even if not reported to medical meetings or journals.

In Britain many units (our own included) continued to ventilate most such patients to an inexorable asystole. It was a harrowing experience for doctors, nurses, and relatives. The problem was discussed informally on several occasions. Not surprisingly little of this gruesome practice ever filtered through to the medical press, but imperceptibly in the early 1970s practice began to change. In 1970 the neurosurgical group at the Salpêtrière, Paris, published an important study showing that in nearly 70 patients with structural brain disease sustained apnoeic coma and absent brainstem reflexes always heralded asystole, despite the fullest possible ventilatory support.[3] Moreover, these clinical signs usually preceded the development of an isoelectric electroencephalogram. A year later the Minnesota criteria were published,[4] and we began to wonder about some of the things we were doing. The publication of the United Kingdom code provided welcome guidance.[5]

Non-drugged patients diagnosed as brain dead by clinical criteria and maintained on ventilator

Series	Year	Patients accepted	Silent electro-encephalograms/electroencephalo-grams obtained	Survivors
Löfsted and von Reis[28]	1959	97	2/2	0
Heiskanen[29]	1964	19	0/0	0
Goulon[30]	1966	1	0/1	0
Lindgren et al[31]	1968	35	27/35	0
Becker et al.[32]	1970	15	6/?*	0
Gaches et al[3]	1970	69	2/69	0
Mohandas and Chou[33]	1971	25	3/9	0
Ingvar and Widen[34]	1972	26	26/26	0
Ouaknine[35]	1975	42	32/32	0
Walker and Molinari[36]	1975	141	130/141	0
Rappaport et al[37]	1978	3	0/1	0
Ayim and Clark[38]	1979	30	3/10	0
Hicks and Torda[39]	1979	21	18/21	0
Ashwal and Schneider[40]	1979	5	0/5	0
Kaste et al[41]	1979	12	?/8*	0
Powner and Fromm[42]	1979	182	164/182	0
Namazie[43]	1980	10	2/2	0
Jennett et al[44]	1981	326	67/70	0
Jørgensen[45]	1981	70	Not stated*	0
Caronna and Plum[46]	1981	34	1/10	0
Rowland et al[47]	1983	10	0/	0
Goulon[48]	1984	23	23/23	0
Nishimura and Sugi[49]	1984	12	Not stated*	0
Ogata et al[50]	1986	45	Not stated*	0
Yoshioka et al[51]	1986	16	Not stated*	0
Hung and Tsai[52]	1986	41	Not stated*	0
Takeuchi et al[53]	1987	552	464/467	0
Total		1862	964/1106	0

*Excluded from totals (data incomplete)

Note—The number of cases (from each reported series) accepted for analysis in this table is often smaller than the totals mentioned in the series themselves. Despite the development of asystole in all cases some of the patients did not, in our opinion, fulfil adequate clinical criteria of brain death, and some of the series include cases of drug intoxication. An additional 92 cases from two further series[54][55] have not been included (although clinically brainstem dead and ventilated to asystole) because it was impossible to ascertain exactly what proportion of these cases was due to structural brain disease. The table deliberately underrepresents the relevant material.

Confidence about withdrawing ventilation was gained only gradually. For instance, over 19 years the proportion of brain dead patients with head injury in Cambridge whose ventilators were electively stopped increased from 6% to 40%.[6] It is still sometimes claimed that there has been no proper "controlled trial" to assess the prognostic value of clinical signs of brainstem death.[7] It is difficult to envisage what the two groups of such a trial might consist of, but it is important to examine the damaging claim that doctors do not really know what happens when they persist in the macabre farce of ventilation after having diagnosed brainstem death. Over 1800 such cases have in fact been published, the second largest series being from three neurosurgical centres in the United Kingdom itself.[6] These cases must comprise only a small minority of those observed over the years around the world. Asystole was the invariable outcome. The table seeks to bring together this scattered material.

One of the main criticisms of codes based on the clinical identification of a dead brainstem is that they could result in diagnoses of death in some patients who might still show some electroencephalographic activity at maximum amplification.[8] It has been emphasised that "the prediction of a fatal outcome is not a valid criterion for the accuracy of standards designed to determine that death has already occurred."[9] We take this to mean that predicting someone is going to die is not the same as saying he or she is already dead. Superficially, this sounds unexceptionable. But it has meaning only if the words "fatal outcome," "dead," and "death" are unquestioningly (and perhaps even reflexly) used in a doubly traditional sense — that is, either as synonyms for "asystole" or as shorthand for the eventual development of an "isoelectric" electroencephalographic pattern characterised (in 1969) as "no activity over 2 µV when recording from scalp electrode pairs 10 or more centimetres apart, with interelectrode resistances of under 10 000 ohms (or impedance under 6000 ohms)."

If one rejects these premises and believes that a person is dead when he or she has irreversibly and as a result of a single event lost both the capacity for consciousness and the capacity to breathe spontaneously, this kind of "critique" assumes a different dimension. It is reduced to the trite conclusion that if a dead brainstem heralds asystole (or the imminent extinction of the electroencephalogram) the differing notions of death are doomed to converge. The words doctors use are indeed important.[10]

of "structural brain damage." One would then need to ascertain how many (if any) of the cases attributed to hypoxia were still showing ultimately reversible brainstem areflexia many hours after their cardiorespiratory arrests. The United Kingdom code *specifically* warns about premature testing of such cases for possible brainstem death. Alleged British survivors of the conditions stipulated in the United Kingdom code were in a different category[21]: they proved to be phantom rabbits conjured out of a phantom hat.[22]

In 1982 American neurologists returned to their critique of the notion that clinical criteria are enough to diagnose brain death.[10 23] They were then referring to a little known document from the National Institutes of Health which mentions three patients seen in the American Collaborative Study of 1971–3.[24] The patients had primary brainstem haemorrhages and soon came to necropsy (which makes one wonder why they were being mentioned). All three had been in "apnoeic" coma. Two had brainstem areflexia (the third had not had his brainstem reflexes fully tested). One patient showed a return of respiration for 24 hours before death. This is the gist of the evidence against the United Kingdom code. But was this single patient ever genuinely apnoeic in the first instance? When previously challenged in 1978 as to how "absence of overriding the respirator for 15 minutes" could be construed as apnoea, the first author of the above report had himself agreed that this was an unsatisfactory test.[25] *Parturiunt montes; nascetur ridiculus mus.*

The existence of other cases is also hinted at but without references, precise specification of cause, or documentation about complicating factors. Anecdotes of this kind — and there will doubtless be others — are inevitable when patients are said to be in apnoeic coma without due attention being paid to what the words mean. Leading participants in the American Collaborative Study believed that "clinical judgment must often suffice in the evaluation of apnoea"[26] and, in 1981 were openly admitting that apnoea in the study "was arbitrarily defined."[27]

1 Working Group of Conference of Medical Royal Colleges and their Faculties in United Kingdom. The critera for the diagnosis of brainstem death. *J R Coll Phys (Lond)* 1995; **29**:281–2.
2 Silverman D, Masland R L, Saunders M G, Schwab R S. Irreversible coma associated with electrocerebral silence. *Neurology* 1970; **20**:525–33.
3 Gaches J, Caliscan A, Findji F, *et al*. Contribution à l'étude du coma dépassé et de la mort cérébrale (étude de 71 cas). *Sem Hôp Paris* 1970; **46**:1487–97.
4 Mohandas A, Chou SN. Brain death. A clinical and pathological study. *J Neurosurg* 1971; **35**:211–18.
5 Working Group of Conferences of Medical Royal Colleges and their Faculties in the United Kingdom. Diagnosis of death. *BMJ* 1976; **ii**:1187–8.
6 Jennett B, Gleave J, Wilson P. Brain deaths in three neurosurgical units. *BMJ* 1981; **282**:533–9.
7 Evans DW. Questioning view of heart transplants. The Times 1982; Sept 13.
8 Walker A E, Molinari GF. Criteria of cerebral death. *Trans Am Neurol Assoc* 1975; **100**:29–35.
9 Molinari GF. Review of clinical critera of brain death. *Ann N Y Acad Sci* 1978; **315**:62–9.
10 Molinari GF. Brain death, irreversible coma, and words doctors use. *Neurology* 1982; **32**:400–2.
11 Jørgensen EO. Spinal man after brain death. *Acta Neurochir (Wien)* 1973; **28**:259–73.
12 Parisi JE, Kim RC, Collins GH, Hillfinger MF. Brain death with prolonged somatic survival. *N Engl J Med* 1982; **306**:14–16.
13 Neagle CE. Brain death with prolonged somatic survival. *N Engl J Med* 1982; **306**:1361–3.
14 Capron AM, Lynn J. Brain death with prolonged somatic survival. *N Engl J Med* 1982; **306**:1362.
15 Yoshioka T, Sugimoto H, Uenishi M, *et al*. Prolonged haemodynamic maintenance by the administration of vasopressin and epinephrine in brain death: a clinical study. *Neurosurgery* 1986; **18**:565–7.
16 Pallis C. Medicine and the media. *BMJ* 1980; **281**:1029.
17 Korein J. Diagnosis of brain death. *BMJ* 1980; **281**:1424.
18 Hughes J. *A question of life and death*. London: BBC Television, 1981. (Transcript of programme shown on 19 Feb.).
19 Bennett DR. Brain death. *Lancet* 1981; **i**:106.
20 Pallis C, MacGillivray B. Brain death. *Lancet* 1981; **i**:223.
21 Paul R. The brain death debate. *Lancet* 1981; **i**:502.
22 Paul R. Survival after brain death: withdrawal of allegation. *Lancet* 1981; **i**:677.
23 Hughes JR. Guidelines for determination of death. *Neurology* 1982 **32**:682–3.
24 Allen N, Burkholder J D, Molinari G F, Comisctoni V. *Clinical criteria of brain death*. Bethesda: National Institutes of Health, 1980; 77–147. (NINCDS Monograph No 24, NIH Publ No 81–2286.)
25 Allen N, Burkholder J. Clinical criteria of brain death. *Ann N Y Acad Sci* 1978; **315**:70–96.
26 Korein J. Neurology and cerebral death: definitions and differential diagnosis. *Transactions of the American Neurological Association* 1975; **100**:210–2.
27 Walker AE. *Cerebral death*. 2nd ed. Baltimore: Urban and Schwarzenberg, 1981.
28 Löfsted SL, von Reis G. *Opuscula Med* 1959; **4**:345.
29 Heiskanen O. Cerebral circulatory arrest caused by acute increase of intracranial pressure. *Acta Neurol Scand* 1964; **40(suppl 7)**:7–52.
30 Goulon M. Le coma dépassé et les comas avec sidération végétative transitoire. *Marseille Chir* (1966) 18.
31 Lindgren S, Petersen I, Zwetnow N. Prediction of death in serious brain damage. *Acta Chir Scand* 1968; **134**:406–16.
32 Becker DP, Robert CM, Nelson JR, *et al*. An evaluation of the definition of cerebral death. *Neurol* 1970; **20**:459–62.
33 Mohandas A, Chou SN. Brain death. A clinical and pathological study. *J Neurosurg* 1971; **35**: 211–8.
34 Ingvar DH, Widen L. Hjärndöd-Sammanfattning av ett Symposium. *Läkartidningen* 1972; **69**:3804–14.
35 Ouaknine GE. Bedside procedures in the diagnosis of brain death. *Resuscitation* 1975; **4**:159–77.
36 Walker AE, Molinari GF. Criteria of cerebral death. *Transactions of the American Neurological Association* 1975; **100**:29–35.
37 Rappaport ZH, Brinker RA, Rovit RL. Evaluation of brain death by contrast-enhanced computerised cranial tomography.*Neurosurgery* 1978; **2**:230–2.
38 Ayim EN, Clark GPM. Brain death: experience in an intensive care unit. *East Afr Med J* 1979; **56**:571–6.
39 Hicks RG, Torda TA. The vestibulo-ocular (caloric) reflex in the diagnosis of cerebral death. *Anaesth Intensive Care* 1979; **7**:169–73.
40 Ashwal S, Schneider S. Failure of electroencephalography to diagnose brain death in comatose children. *Ann Neurol* 1979; **6**:512–7.
41 Kaste M, Hillbom M, Palo J. Diagnosis and management of brain death. *BMJ* 1979; **i**:525–7.
42 Powner DJ, Fromm GH. The electroencephalogram in the determination of brain death. *N Engl J Med* 1979; **300**:502.
43 Namazie M. Diagnosis and management of brain death. *Med J Malaysia* 1980; **34**:363–7.
44 Jennett B, Gleave J, Wilson P. Brain deaths in three neurosurgical units. *BMJ* 1981; **282**:533–9.
45 Jørgensen EO. Brain death: retrospective surveys. *Lancet* 1981; **i**:378–9.
46 Caronna JJ, Plum F. In: Plum F, Posner JB, eds. *The diagnosis of stupor and coma*. 3rd ed. Philadelphia: Davis, 1980.
47 Rowland TW, Donnelly JH, Jackson AH, Jamroz SB. Brain death in the pediatric intensive care unit. A clinical definition. *Am J Dis Child* 1983; **137**:547.
48 Goulon M. *International Critical Care Digest* 1984; **3**:23.
49 Nishimura N, Sugi T. Circulatory support with sympathetic amines in brain death. *Resuscitation* 1984; **12**:25.
50 Ogata J, Yutani C, Imakita M, Ueda H. Autolysis of the granular layer of the

cerebellar cortex in brain death. *Acta Neuropathol (Berl)* 1986; **70**:75–8.

51 Yoshioka T, Sugimoto H, Uenishi M, *et al*. Prolonged haemodynamic maintenance by the combined administration of vasopressin and epinephrine in brain death: a clinical study. *Neurosurgery* 1986; **18**:565.

52 Hung TP, Tsai TT. *J Formos Med Assoc* 1986; **85**:514.

53 Takeuchi K, Takeshita H, Takakura K, *et al*. Evolution of criteria for determi-

nation of brain death in Japan. *Acta Neurochir (Wien)* 1987; **87**:93.

54 Ibe K. Clinical and pathophysiological aspects of intravital brain death. *Electroencephalogr Clin Neurophysiol* 1971; **30**:272.

55 Korein J, Maccario M. On the diagnosis of cerebral death: a prospective study of 55 patients to define irreversible coma. *Clin Electroencephalogr* 1971; **2**:178–99.

8 CEREBRAL BLOOD FLOW, ELECTROENCEPHALOGRAPHY, AND OTHER DIAGNOSTIC METHODS

There seems to be a tendency in medical practice throughout the developed world, and indeed the developing world, to base the diagnosis of brain death on either the United Kingdom code or the United States guidelines. Clinical testing in both countries is virtually identical: both practices demand that the patient be in deep apnoeic coma and without brainstem reflexes; currently demand proper documentation of the apnoea; and now emphasise the importance of a definite diagnosis, although the concept of "preconditions" and "exclusions" is not as widely spoken about in the United States as it is in the United Kingdom. An apparent substitute for this is the emphasis in the United States on "confirmatory" (usually instrumental) corroboration of the diagnosis.

Many institutions and countries worldwide insist on these allegedly objective tests to establish that the brain has ceased to function. This seems to stem from reluctance to accept, or perhaps just unfamiliarity with, the conceptual difference between "death of the whole brain" and "death of the brain as a whole" — that is, brainstem death. In some countries doctors are also under considerable legislative or public pressure to "prove" a lack of all supratentorial activity. Such an approach fails to appreciate the truly massive nature of the supratentorial pathology required to produce irreversible loss of all brainstem function, or the supratentorial implications, in terms of irreversible loss of the capacity for consciousness, of primary brainstem lesions large enough to cause both apnoea and loss of all the brainstem reflexes.

The pressure for "objective" tests generally takes the form of an insistence on the instrumental demonstration of "electrocerebral silence" or a "blocked cerebral circulation," or both. This has led to sustained efforts to discover ever more sophisticated tests for confirming whole brain death. Most such tests seek to prove lack of blood flow to both supratentorial areas and to the brainstem, which is then equated with whole brain death.

If we accept that such tests will confirm alleged brain death, what is their reliability? How reproducible are they? How complex are they to administer and interpret?

> ## Methods used to "confirm" brain death
>
> - Angiography (contrast and radionuclide)
> - Doppler ultrasonography
> - Magnetic resonance imaging
> - Brainstem auditory evoked potentials
> - Metabolic and hormonal markers
> - Electroencephalography

Tests for demonstrating absent blood flow
Contrast medium angiography

Throughout the 1950s and 1960s neuroradiologists repeatedly showed the phenomenon of cerebral circulatory arrest. It was commonly found in patients with head injury, cerebral haemorrhage, or other structural brain lesions, particularly if there had been respiratory complications. The basis of such a finding was the reduction of cerebral perfusion as a result of cerebral oedema or the loss of cerebrovascular autoregulation, or both. Tentorial pressure cones also contributed. The main problem was that it was not uncommon for there to be vertebral flow without carotid flow and vice versa. It was also found that it was possible for there to be electroencephalographic activity after demonstration of "absent cerebral circulation."[1 2] Again, the reduction of intracranial pressure by removing a haematoma or by hyperventilation and the administration of mannitol sometimes resulted in the restoration of blood flow. The question was how "blocked" did the cerebral circulation have to be before you could conclude that the whole brain was dead? In a review of the problem Bricolo *et al* reported patients with non-filling and silent electroencephalograms who had "clear signs of cerebral life" and the reversal of no flow situations after removal of a tumour or haematoma or hyperventilation.[3] In infants and the newborn, in whom the diagnosis of brain death is notoriously difficult, digital subtraction angiography has been suggested. A report indicates it may be of value in demonstrating lack of cerebral flow.[4] Nevertheless, these techniques have considerable drawbacks and better methods are continually being sought.

Isotope angiography

Isotope angiography (radionuclide cerebral perfusion scintigraphy) is based on the assumption that cerebral blood flow at levels too low to be detected by the technique is insufficient to maintain the metabolic requirements of the brain. Radionuclide imaging has been shown in many studies to be capable of equalling conventional angiography of supratentorial structures, especially if technetium-99m hexamethyl-propylenamine oxime (99mTc-HMPAO) is used, and the results have equated well with clinical evidence of brainstem death.[5–8] It should be noted that it was discovered at an early stage that isotope angiography was not suitable for demonstrating the vertebrobasilar vasculature. Hence, the demonstration of brainstem blood flow could not be relied on with this technique. If studies with single positron emission computed tomography (SPECT) are carried out as well then flow in both infratentorial and supratentorial structures can be examined. Nevertheless, in those studies where some residual flow coexisted with clinical evidence of brainstem areflexia, all patients developed asystole. The primary use of the tests is in "both the mitigation of uncertainty due to factors interfering with the clinical examination and in expediting the correct diagnosis of brain death." Under United Kingdom criteria, of course, the mere fact of uncertainty in clinical examination would invalidate any tests for brainstem death. However, the tests suffer from the same drawbacks as contrast angiography — raised intracranial pressure will interfere with the distribution of isotopes.

Transcranial Doppler flow imaging

If arteries supplying the brain can be examined by ultrasonic means by using Doppler techniques, flow through relevant arteries should be assessable. It has been found that in "brain dead" patients there is absent or reversed diastolic flow or small early systolic spikes in more than one intracranial artery.[9][10] Transcranial Doppler methods will show flow through the middle cerebral and basilar arteries. In one study 140 patients, 11 of whom were believed to be brain dead, underwent Doppler ultrasonography before formal brainstem testing.[11] Those showing retrograde flow or just sharp systolic peaks proved to have areflexic brainstems. They all developed asystole. Patients in whom flow occurred throughout the cardiac cycle and who failed to satisfy the brainstem tests all survived. The results of this study agreed completely with angiography and clinical testing. Other studies have given similar results.

Magnetic resonance imaging

Flow sensitive gradient-echo sequences on magnetic resonance imaging (MRI) can demonstrate the absence of flow in the cerebral circulation.[12] The future place of this technique is still uncertain. As the scanners are not bedside instruments there are major logistical problems of moving ill patients and maintaining their ventilation in the confines of an MRI tube. The use of intravenous phosphorus (P^{31}) with magnetic resonance imaging showed a complete absence of ATP and an intense inorganic phosphate signal, suggesting that flow was absent.[13] This would also imply that cerebral metabolism had been reduced below that necessary for cerebral survival.

Brainstem auditory evoked potentials

The application of brainstem auditory evoked potentials has been the subject of a great deal of research. Much of this has been directed at efforts to determine levels of consciousness. This method has been widely studied in determining alterations in brainstem activity in, for instance, anaesthesia. It has the advantage of being a bedside technique. In essence acoustic stimuli are applied and the resulting activity of the brainstem is recorded with modified electroencephalographic techniques. The pattern of waves on the tracing and the presence or absence of some or all waves are directly related to levels of brainstem activity. The results are not affected by sedative drugs so the technique can be used in those patients in whom residual drug effects may be influencing diagnosis as when the administration of barbiturate is being used as part of the "treatment" of the cerebral condition. It is important to remember that previous deafness can render the test useless and that the presence of a petrous fracture must be excluded. This test is potentially useful.[14][15] An investigation of 33 patients in Ankara with brainstem auditory evoked potentials and radionuclide and brain perfusion studies showed a close correlation in the results.[16] All those patients with absent brainstem auditory evoked potentials showed a "blocked cerebral circulation" and this, added to the clinical findings, resulted in a diagnosis of brain death. Similar results have been reported elsewhere.[17] Anoxia may cause a reversible loss of brainstem auditory evoked potentials components.[18] Indeed in some of the reports many of the patients investigated would not have satisfied the United Kingdom clinical preconditions for brainstem death.

A further use of brainstem auditory evoked potentials is to help with diagnosis of brainstem death in those patients who have been managed with barbiturate infusions as part of the "treatment" of their coma. It has been shown that the technique can demonstrate brainstem activity (or lack of it) under these conditions. It can certainly prove helpful in those cases when residual sedative drugs may confuse the issue.

Metabolic and hormonal markers

Great efforts have been made to determine whether the presence or absence of various biochemical markers could be of value in the diagnosis of brain death. Thus thyrotropin releasing hormone may be used to demonstrate lack of thyrotropin and prolactin secretion in brain dead patients.[19] It has been asserted that changes in levels of hypothalamic hormones, the presence or absence of glucose metabolism, and the production of excess lactate are relevant in determining brain death. Reduction in the concentration of antidiuretic hormone and the subsequent diabetes insipidus are a common occurrence in severe brain damage, but estimation of the concentrations of the relevant hormones has proved disappointing prognostically. Positron emission tomography has been used to show lack of glucose metabolism in the apparently dead brain. The measurement of cerebral venous oxygen saturation in a severely brain damaged patient by using jugular bulb catheterisation showed a characteristic dip and rise at the point of loss of brainstem auditory evoked potentials and electroencephalographic silence.[20] Like so many investigations the results of most of these tests are, at best, equivocal and require highly skilled interpreters.

It is evident from the multiplicity of tests that have been devised that none give unequivocal answers. Many are performed on patients who would not pass the first hurdle if assessed by the United Kingdom criteria. It would seem pointless to indulge in such tests for brain(stem) death if, for instance, the cause of the coma is not known, or if the patient is still breathing or exhibiting posturing. Yet it is still done. We might well ask the question posed below about the electroencephalogram. What do the tests tell us that we could not establish by properly conducted clinical examination after rigorous exclusions?

The electroencephalogram
The conceptual argument

The main argument about the electroencephalogram is conceptual, not technical. To what overall concept of death does the electroencephalographic criterion (of electrocerebral silence) relate? Whether they realise it or not the advocates and the detractors of electroencephalography are pursuing different objectives, related to different concepts of death. The former are seeking to diagnose the biological "death of the whole brain" — that is, the death of most, if not all, brain cells. With this objective in mind the scalp electroencephalogram may be considered relevant (provided you keep in mind that it is quite incapable of achieving the desired end). Those who claim that the electroencephalogram is irrelevant are seeking to diagnose death of the brain as a functional unit (death of the "brain as a whole"). They do this by concentrating on what allows the brain to function as a unit: the brainstem. In pursuit of that objective the electroencephalogram is indeed irrelevant. Recording an electroencephalogram from the scalp is not testing a brainstem function.

How important, in practice, is the difference between the two approaches? An important study carried out at the Salpêtrière Hospital in Paris over 20 years ago showed that when apnoeic coma and absent brainstem reflexes occurred in a context of structural brain disease minor residual electroencephalographic activity was common but never persisted.[21] In nearly all cases no electroencephalogram could be recorded after 48 hours.

The table seeks to make a different but equally relevant point. It too deals with patients suffering from structural brain disease, contrasting the prognostic implications of clinically dead brainstems (in patients with remnants of electroencephalographic activity) with the prognostic implications of "isoelectric" electroencephalograms (in patients with residual clinical signs of brainstem function).[22] All patients with potentially reversible causes

Prognostic significance of brainstem signs (structural brain lesions, no drug induced cases)

No of cases	Brainstem areflexia	Apnoea	Electro-encephalogram	Aystole within days
>1000	All	All	Isoelectric	All
147	All	All	Some residual activity	All
16	None	None	Isoelectric	None

of brainstem dysfunction (such as drugs and metabolic disturbances) were excluded in this survey. Over 1000 subjects were identified who had apnoeic coma, brainstem areflexia, and an "isoelectric" electroencephalogram. All developed asystole within days. A further 147 cases were identified, with brainstem areflexia and apnoea, in whom there was some residual electroencephalographic activity. Again, all developed asystole within a few days. Like the first group, they also had dead brainstems. The conclusion seems to be that, irrespective of what the electroencephalogram may show, a clinically dead brainstem always heralds asystole. A further 16 well

---

Sources of electro-encephalographic artefacts

Idiomuscular potentials
Pulse
Electrocardiography
Ballistocardiography
Pacemaker
Dialysis machine
Respirator artefacts:
   Head movements
   Ventilation tube vibrations
People touching the bed
People passing the bed
Fluid dripping from patient
Fluid dripping into patient
Sphygmomanometer
Hiccough
Shivering

---

documented case reports were found of patients who had isoelectric electroencephalograms (strictly defined) but some residual brainstem function. None of these developed asystole. Again this is not surprising: parts of their brainstems were still functioning.

The technical argument

The technical argument has centred on the fact that an intensive care unit is about the most hostile environment imaginable for trying to record "electrocerebral silence." Many electroencephalograms in these circumstances show multiple artefacts which may be bizarre and difficult to identify and locate. If the attendant is wearing nylon clothing static electricity may generate false signals. Electromagnetic disturbances from call systems may also generate confusing information. But apart from artefacts some experts have argued that it is intrinsically impossible to record a genuinely isoelectric electroencephalogram at an amplification of $2 \mu V/mm$ because this is approaching the noise level of even the most sensitive apparatus.[23] To exclude cerebral activity of just over this magnitude (in a noisy trace inevitably contaminated by signals several times larger) is certainly a major demand not always achievable.

Anyway, does an isoelectric tracing from the scalp imply electrocerebral silence, as is so often implied? What about signals generated in the depths of the sulci or by the basal cortex? Why are the advocates of electroencephalography not requesting traces from pharyngeal or sphenoidal electrodes? And what about attenuation of signals en route to the scalp? Even at normal voltage such attenuation may be considerable. But even if the whole of the cortex could be shown to be electrically silent (which is impossible) would it mean that every cell in the brain was dead? There have been cases where thalamic probing has shown persistent neuronal discharges in the presence of an isoelectric electroencephalogram.[24] Electroencephalography therefore does not test cerebral function with the rigour demanded by the concept of death of the whole brain. If those who accept this concept were logical they would have to drill burrholes and probe with depth electrodes before diagnosing a totally dead brain.

There is a final facet to the technical critique. The electroencephalogram is often said to be "objective." This is not so. In the American Collaborative Study special efforts were made to identify artefacts in the records, yet about 6% of 2256 electroencephalograms were classified as unsatisfactory because of technical difficulties.[25] Discordance between those interpreting the records was put at only 3%, which is exceptionally good. There is no sharp end point, as recordable electroencephalographic activity gradually submerges into noise. A German survey showed that the reliability and validity of the electroencephalogram when assessed by and between expert electroencephalographic diagnosticians was low.[26] They admitted that "the limited reliability of the electroencephalogram in the diagnosis of brain death must be accepted." These are not the hallmarks of an "objective" test.

The clinical argument

Those who argue that the electroencephalogram is irrelevant to establishing the presence of a dead brainstem are often misunderstood. They are *not* saying the electroencephalogram is irrelevant to the diagnosis of the condition causing the coma (it may be most useful, for instance, in establishing a diagnosis of hepatic encephalopathy or of herpes simplex encephalitis). Nor are they denying the prognostic value of the electroencephalogram after head injury or acute cerebral anoxia, although even here there is evidence that judiciously directed clinical assessments may provide very reliable prognostic data. There is even evidence that in patients rendered comatose after a cardiac arrest the clinical signs elicited within the first hour may indicate whether the electroencephalogram will remain isoelectric.[27]

There seems to be a difference of opinion among the advocates of the electroencephalogram about its exact purpose. Some believe it to be necessary for ascertaining that unspecified preconditions have been met. Others consider it part of the final testing, an isoelectric trace being deemed the ultimate proof that the brain is dead. Neither attitude is warranted. In patients in deep coma electroencephalography may generate misleading data.[28 29] To those unaware of the pitfalls it may suggest death in patients who may survive. There is a report of a patient being declared dead on the basis of a single electroencephalogram. Conversely, persistent electroencephalographic activity often generates false hope in relation to "beating heart cadavers," doomed to develop asystole because their brainstems are already dead. It has been claimed that to do an electroencephalogram in the clinical context of brainstem death is "reassuring" to the relatives. We believe such recordings are often done to reassure doctors. If the electroencephalogram is recorded in the knowledge (which the relatives do not share) that it is non-contributory this is manipulative behaviour.

In summary, the electroencephalogram relates (inaccurately) to an unformulated (but unacceptable) concept of death. It provides answers of variable reliability to what is widely felt to be the wrong question. This should make it of very doubtful utility for anyone with any concern for intellectual clarity in this field. To the more pragmatically minded the capacity of the electroencephalogram to lead to wrong practical decisions should suggest caution in its use.

The argument about residual sentience

Is there more than atavistic mysticism in the essentially untestable supposition of residual sentience in the isolated forebrain, or in cell aggregates elsewhere in the cortex or deeper structures? Clinical experience offers no support for this notion. Really deep coma, as distinct from stupor or delirium, is always associated with an absence of purposeful response to stimuli and is always followed by profound amnesia, no matter what the cause of the coma. Confusion is engendered by including in discussions about residual sentience and the electroencephalogram a wide variety of different neurological conditions, ranging from the persistent vegetative state to physiological sleep, and including such diverse entities as experiences during the induction of anaesthesia in a normal person and the "locked in" syndrome in a fully conscious individual. The electroencephalographic correlates of such a miscellany will, of course, range from "electrocerebral silence" to normal activity.

The question is sometimes asked whether the small part of the reticular formation situated rostral to the brainstem proper could generate anything remotely resembling a capacity for consciousness. There is little anatomical basis for such an assumption. Current concepts of the reticular formation still emphasise the primacy of the brainstem nuclei. The reticular formation

of the thalamus has predominantly internal connections. It has an important gating role, but there is little to suggest that it has widespread cortical projections, as does the reticular formation of the brainstem.

We do not believe there could be residual sentience above a dead brainstem. But we would ask those who disagree — and who want to be logical about the conclusions to be drawn from their premises — to face up to the scenario of a patient with a dead brainstem, doomed to asystole within a few days, yet showing remnants of electroencephalographic activity (which they equate with residual sentience). Can they conceive of a greater hell than an isolated sentience, aware of its precarious existence, and with no means of expression? Would they anaesthetise such a preparation? Or just sedate it? And might not this further depression of cerebral function, in a patient already in *coma dépassé*, prove to be the last straw?

The problem has, of course, fascinated physiologists and philosophers for generations. With appropriate corrections of time scale, it is the problem of what happens, for a few seconds, in a decapitated head. The following limerick, which could have been written by one of the *tricoteuses* sitting at the foot of the guillotine in Paris in 1793, puts the forbidden question:

> We knit on, too *blasées* to ask it:
> Could the tetraparesis just mask it?
> When the brainstem is dead
> Can the cortex be said
> To tick on, in the head, in the basket?

The cultural argument

Electroencephalograms are, nevertheless, still widely resorted to in the United States and elsewhere in the diagnosis of brain death. Few people are prepared to discuss the cultural (rather than neurological) dimensions of this addiction. Our American colleagues practise in a litigious atmosphere in which "a climate of general public unease about brain death exists, partly engendered by sensational fiction."[30] This legal unease is also at least in part behind many countries' use of electroencephalography. For good or ill, instrumental medicine has taken giant steps forward — often evicting good clinical practice in its wake. Many American jurors have a touchingly naive faith in the supremacy of machines such as the electroencephalograph, do not realise that there is at least a 3% variance in the reading of such records, and are blissfully unaware of the problems of obtaining traces free of artefact at high amplification.

Leading neurologists in the United States readily endorse these doubts about the scientific relevance of the electroencephalogram and emphasise that in the "less legally demanding" conditions of the United Kingdom "it is doubtful that the experienced physician needs the electroencephalogram to tell him that the brain is dead." But, as an American colleague wrote to me, they "have to protect the young people who are educated with them against the malevolent ravages of opportunistic lawyers." They live "in a climate where physicians have been brought to court as potential murderers for having killed an already dead patient." (F Plum, personal communication). Physicians resort to electroencephalograms to "save a great deal of later polemical accusation."

It was suggested in the *Panorama* programme on brain death (13 October 1980) and is still believed in the United

States, that our reluctance in the United Kingdom to use electroencephalography for diagnosing brain death is due to the paucity of such machines in our hospitals. Economics, it was claimed, was a consideration in formulating our code. The paucity of machines is admitted but the implication is unwarranted. As the question of economics has been raised, let us say that we believe it to be relevant to the continued advocacy of instrumental diagnosis in the United States. Vested interests should be openly declared. They rarely are, in either verbal or written discussions on the use of electroencephalography in the diagnosis of death. They should certainly not be confused with physiological principles.

Conclusions

Modern technology in its desperate attempts to save human life has produced an entity widely known as brain death. It has also generated a conceptual crisis: that of knowing — at the simplest, bedside level — whether a patient is alive or dead.

We have argued that the conceptual challenge can and should be met. We must evolve a concept of death that is in keeping with the cultural context of our age and which would in practice enable us to steer a course between "treating the putrefying body as if it were alive, and treating patients who are mentally retarded as if they were dead."[31] The recognition of a dead brainstem is the first step along such a course. In this book we are seeking to show how such a state can be identified clinically and how it relates to an overall concept of death.

The lay public, however, is not on the whole interested in physiological arguments about the reticular formation or in philosophical controversies about the nature of death. People are concerned that their kidneys should not be removed while they are comatose from treatable conditions. The United Kingdom code can give the public absolute reassurance in this respect. It is scentifically sound and clinically foolproof (provided the necessary attention is given to preconditions and exclusions and provided the doctors carrying out the tests are reasonably competent and know what they are doing and why). The whole ethos subtending the code is humane. In practice it will be of help to relatives, nursing staff, and doctors who "may unintentionally find themselves caring for a biological preparation with no other human attributes than physical form."[32]

As if anticipating later developments, Shakespeare had Macbeth proclaim (act III, scene IV) that there was once a time "that when the brains were out, the man would die." The challenge today is a double one: to replace the words "would die" by the words "is dead" — and to be more specific about "the brains being out." The death of the brainstem would surely be enough.

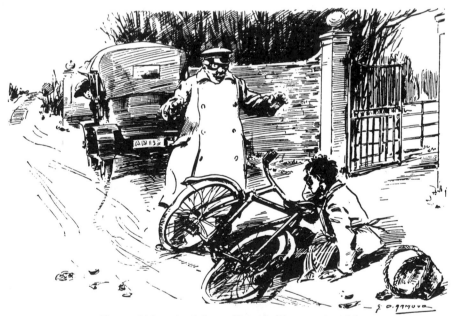

Alarmed Motorist (after collision): "Are you hurt?"
Butcher Boy: "Where's my Kidneys?"

1 Brock M, Fieschi C, Ingvar DH, eds. *Cerebral blood flow*. Berlin: Springer-Verlag, 1969.
2 Ashwal S, Schneider S. Failure of electroenphalography to diagnose brain death in comatose children. *Ann Neurol* 1979; **6**:512–7.
3 Bricolo A, Dalle Ore G, Da Pian R, Benati A, Turella G. In: Fusek, Kunc, eds. *Present limits of neurosurgery*. Prague: Avicenum, 1972.
4 Albertini A, Schonfeld S, Hiatt M, Hegyi T. Digital substraction angiography — a new approach to brain death determination in the newborn. *Pediatr Radiol* 1993; **23**:195–7.
5 Schlake HP, Bottger IG, Grotemeyer KH, Husstedt IW, Brandau W, Schober O. *Intensive Care Medicine* 1992; **18**:76–81.
6 Wilson K, Gordon L, Selby J sr. The diagnosis of brain death with Tc-99m HMPAO. *Clin Nucl Med* 1993; **18**:428–34.
7 Wieler H, Marohl K, Kaiser KP, Klawki P, Frossler H. Tc-99m HMPAO cerebral scintigraphy. A reliable noninvasive method for determination of brain death. *Clin Nucl Med* 1993; **18**:104–9.
8 De la Riva A, Gonzalez FM, Llamas-Elvira JM, Latre JM, Jinenez-Heffernan A, Vidal E, *et al.* Diagnosis of brain death: superiority of perfusion studies with Tc-99m HMPAO over conventional radionuclide cerebral angiography. *Br J Radiol* 1992; **65**:289–94.
9 Petty GW, Mohr JP, Pedley TA, Tatemichi TK, Lennihan L, Duterte DI, *et al.* The role of transcranial Doppler in confirming brain death. *Neurology* 1990; **40**:300-3.
10 Davalos A, Rodriguez-Rago A, Mate G, Molins A, Genis D, Gonzalez JL. Value of the transcranial Doppler examination in the diagnosis of brain death. *Med Clin* 1993; **100**:249–52.
11 Zurynski Y, Dorsch N, Pearson I, Choong R. Transcranial Doppler ultrasound in brain death: experience in 140 patients. *Neurol Res* 1991; **13**:248–52.
12 Jones KM, Barnes PD. MR diagnosis of brain death. *American Journal of Neuroradiology* 1992; **13**:65–6.
13 Aichner F, Felber S, Birbamer G, Luz G, Judmaier W, Schmutzhard E. Magnetic resonance: a non-invasive approach to metabolism, circulation, and morphology in human brain death. *Ann Neurol* 1992; **32**:507–11.
14 Firsching R, Reinhold A F, Wilhelms S, Buchholz F. Brain death: practicability of evoked potentials. *Neurosurg Rev* 1992; **15**:249–54.
15 Guerit M. Evoked potentials: a safe brain-death confirmatory tool? *Eur J Med* 1992; **1**:233–43.
16 Erbengi A, Erbengi G, Cataltepe O, Topcu M, Erbas B, Aras T. Brain death: determination with brainstem evoked potentials and radionuclide isotope studies. *Acta Neurochir (Wien)* 1991; **112**:118–25.

17 Palma V, Guadagnino M. Evoked potentials in brain death. A critical review. *Acta Neurologica* 1992; **14**:363–68.

18 Schmitt B, Simma B, Burger R, Dumermuth G. Resuscitation after severe hypoxia in a young child: temporary isoelectric EEG and loss of brainstem auditory evoked potentials components. *Intensive Care Medicine* 1993; **19**:420–2.

19 Imberti R, Filisetti P, Preseglio I, Mapelli A, Spriano P. Confirmation of brain death utilizing thyrotropin-releasing hormone stimulation test. *Neurosurgery* 1990; **27**:167.

20 Hantson P, Mahieu P. Usefulness of cerebral venous monitoring through jugular bulb catheterisation for the diagnosis of brain death [Letter]. *Intensive Care Medicine* 1992; **18**:59.

21 Gaches J, Calisan A, Findji F, *et al*. Contribution à l'étude du coma dépassé et de la mort cérébrale (étude de 71 cas). *Sem Hôp Paris* 1970; **46**:1487–97.

22 Pallis C. Prognostic value of brainstem lesion. *Lancet* 1981; i:379.

23 Jørgensen EO. Requirements for recording the EEG at high sensitivity in suspected brain death. *Electroencephalogr Clin Neurophysiol* 1974; **36**:65–9.

24 Carbonell J, Carrascosa G, Diersen S, *et al*. Some electrophysiological observations in a case of deep coma secondary to cardiac arrest. *Electroencephalogr Clin Neurophysiol* 1963; **15**:520–5.

25 Bennett D R. The EEG in determination of brain death. *Ann N Y Acad Sci* 1978; **315**:110–9.

26 Buchner H, Schuchardt V. Reliability of electroencephalogram in the diagnosis of brain death. *Eur Neurol* 1990; **30**:138–41.

27 Jørgensen EO, Meichow-Møller A. Natural history of global and critical brain ischaemia. II. EEG and neurological signs in patients remaining unconscious after cardiopulmonary resuscitation. *Resuscitation* 1981; **9**:155–74.

28 Hughes J R. Limitations of the EEG in coma and brain death. *Ann N Y Acad Sci* 1978; **315**:121–36.

29 Pallis C, MacGillivray B. Brain death and the EEG. *Lancet* 1980; ii:1085–6.

30 Sweet W H. Brain death. *N Engl J Med* 1978; **299**:410–2.

31 Veatch R M. The definition of death: ethical, philosophical and policy confusion. *Ann NY Acad Sci* 1978; **315**:307–21.

32 Pearson J, Korein J, Braunstein P. Morphology of defectively perfused brains in patients with persistent extracranial circulation. *Ann NY Acad Sci* 1978; **315**:265–71.

9   THE POSITION IN THE UNITED STATES AND ELSEWHERE

In the early 1970s an American Collaborative Study was set up under the sponsorship of the National Institutes of Neurological and Communicative Disorders and Stroke. Nine centres took part. The study was designed to "formulate a set of criteria that would identify a dead brain in an otherwise living body."[1] The results emerged piecemeal over the next decade in a series of publications dealing with the clinical, pathological, toxicological, and electroencephalographic findings. The wide scatter of the most relevant data made access difficult. Further difficulties arose because different centres in the collaborative study did not use words in the same way. This is shown most clearly in relation to "cerebral death." One active participant urged that the term be used to describe "irreversible destruction of the (intracranial) components above the tentorium."[2] Such a definition would clearly exclude a dead brainstem and suggests a vegetative state. But the coordinator of the study (and author of its main publications) used the words "cerebral death" to denote something quite different and more general — namely, the irreversible cessation of all nervous activity "within the intracranial cavity."[3] This second concept clearly includes a dead brainstem. It describes what most people mean by "whole brain death." A summary statement of the Collaborative Study's findings was published in 1977. If any document can be said to have reflected a substantial segment of opinion in the United States about brain death (before July 1981) it is this.[1] A detailed critique of the collaborative study's findings and methodology has been published elsewhere.[4]

The main difference between the United Kingdom and early American approaches to brain death lay in the concept of the necessary preconditions. In the United Kingdom we placed emphasis on strictly defined preconditions of irremediable structural brain damage and on excluding potentially reversible causes of brainstem dysfunction. In the American Collaborative Study the common clinical causes of brain death were listed as including "drug intoxication or overdose, and metabolic coma."[5] These are potentially reversible causes of neurological disturbance, and, although they may well result in irreversible brain damage, the United Kingdom code specifically warns against considering the diagnosis of brainstem death in patients with such conditions. However, we have not always practised what we preach, and this has left us open to justified criticism from the United States.[6]

Clinical testing was similar in the two countries. Both practices demanded that the patient be in unresponsive coma and without brainstem reflexes (often referred to as "cephalic" reflexes in the American publications). Both practices demanded apnoea, although until the early 1980s this was much more strictly defined in the United Kingdom than in the United States. But in many institutions in the United States (partly as a result of the lack of specification of strict preconditions) there was a

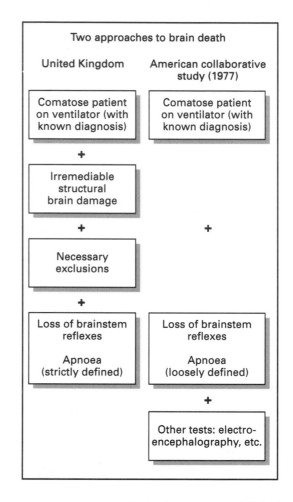

demand for further "objective" tests to establish that the brain had ceased to function. The first and most widely used was of course electroencephalography. Other techniques sought to establish that there was no significant cerebral blood flow. These techniques have also been described in chapter 8 and have been discussed in detail in a previous publication.[4] Meanwhile, simple clinical testing at the bedside has held its own. No adequately documented report of a patient fulfilling the United Kingdom criteria and either recovering consciousness or failing to develop asystole has been published.

Other countries

Different developments were meanwhile taking place elsewhere. At the end of 1979 the renal transplant organisations in 40 countries were questioned by the departments of surgery of the University of Chicago and of the Albert Einstein College of Medicine, New York, and by the department of neurology at the Hennepin County Medical Center, Minneapolis.[7] Neurosurgical societies were also questioned.[3] We have tabulated updated information concerning the legal status of brain

The position in the United States and elsewhere

In Germany, criteria of brain death published in 1982 had already made the useful distinction between primarily intracranial and primarily extracranial causes of the condition. The publication of "third generation criteria" in 1987 was to make further distinctions between primary supratentorial and primary infratentorial lesions.[9] Under certain conditions "the extinction of evoked potentials" could establish the loss of brainstem function and "might offer an alternative" to an isoelectric electroencephalogram or the demonstration of a blocked cerebral circulation. Overall, however, the medical regulatory body (Bundesärzteskammer) currently insists on the use of electroencephalography or flow detection methods to determine brain death after brainstem reflexes have been shown to be absent.[10]

In Italy, there is a requirement for "instrumental techniques" to confirm clinical findings.[11] A new law (No 582) was promulgated in 1994. Clinical findings indicating a non-functioning brainstem are required, but an electroencephalogram is still mandatory. Assessment of cerebral blood flow is still required in children under the age of 1 year, in the presence of pharmacological or metabolic factors which might affect clinical evaluation, and in cases where the clinical evaluation, for whatever reason, cannot properly be carried out. In Scandinavia, criteria for brainstem death were first accepted in Finland in 1971, Sweden in 1988 and Denmark in 1990. The

Basis for diagnosis of brain death

Country	Clinical tests	Electro-encephalo-graphy required	Flow studies required	Brainstem auditory evoked potentials
Australia	+			
Belgium	+			
Canada	+			
Colombia	+			
Finland	+			
Greece	+			
Hungary	+			
India	+			
Ireland	+			
New Zealand	+			
Puerto Rico	+			
Saudi Arabia	+			
South Africa	+			
Taiwan	+			
South Korea	+			
United Kingdom	+			
Uruguay	+			
Austria	+	+		
Brazil	+	+		
Cuba	+	+		
Denmark	+	+		
France	+	+		
Norway	+		+	
Peru	+	+		
Portugal	+	+		
Spain	+	+		
Sweden	+	+		
Switzerland	+	+		
Thailand	+	+		
Venezuela	+	+		
Argentina	+	+ or	+ or	+
Chile	+	+ or	+	
Czech Republic	+	+ or	+	
Germany	+	+ or	+ or	+
Italy	+	+ or	+ or	+
Turkey	+	+ or	+ or	+
United States	+	instrumental testing 'not mandatory' (1995)[39]		

death (and about the tests currently required to establish the diagnosis) in various parts of the world.

All the countries responding to the 1979 questionnaire demanded apnoeic coma and absent brainstem reflexes as integral components of the definition of brain death. Most countries which specified preconditions of structural brain disease did not require additional instrumental tests. Countries which did not specify preconditions — that is, where brain death could be diagnosed in patients suffering from severe drug intoxication, metabolic coma, and so on — required either one or two electroencephalograms, separated by variable periods of time, or one or more angiograms (to show a blocked cerebral circulation), or both electroencephalograms and angiograms.

The situation today varies widely. It has least changed in France, where the concept of *coma dépassé* triggered all subsequent discussion. The *Circulaire Jeanneney* (a document issued by the Ministry of Social Affairs on 24 April 1968) became incorporated in a law (the *loi Caillavet*) in December 1976. The 1968 circular had stipulated that what was needed to diagnose death on neurological grounds were "concordant proofs" (clinical and electroencephalographic) concerning the "irreversibility of lesions incompatible with life." Among the clinical requirements were "dilated pupils, complete hypotonia, and the abolition of all reflexes." A 1986 review suggested that aging precept and current practice were beginning to diverge.[8] This is probably inevitable when the law seeks to "freeze" medical concepts, confining them to what prevailed at earlier points in time.

The position in the United States and elsewhere

Swedish road to consensus proved difficult but informative, the Danish particularly bumpy.[12-14]

In both Spain and Portugal, brain death has legal status, but the diagnosis requires EEG "confirmation." The Greek code, published in March 1985, closely mirrors that in the United Kingdom. No electroencephalography is required. The Swiss code is uniquely detailed. In May 1983 the country's Senate approved new directives for the definition and diagnosis of death.[15] These insisted that in testing for brain death firm pressure be applied over the emergence point of the second division of the trigeminal. They also specified not only a target $Paco_2$ for the disconnection test (6.65 kPa — 59 mm Hg) but an arterial pH of "less than 7.4." Two isoelectric electroencephalograms at 24 hours' interval were said to be diagnostically useful "in some cases of metabolic coma." An excellent review, in German, evaluates the guidelines currently prevailing in Germany, Austria, and Switzerland.[16] Hungary passed a law in 1988 explicitly recognising that brainstem death was legally death. No electroencephalography was required. Surprisingly, in Holland, traditionally a forward-looking and liberal country, electroencephalography or angiography is required in all brainstem dead patients who are to become organ donors, even those who fulfil the preconditions and brainstem death criteria (I R de Jong, personal communication 1994). Poland was unusual. Although brain death was accepted, its logical extension (the concept of what we have called a "beating heart cadaver") was not. Brain death was not unequivocally equated with death. Brain death warranted withdrawal of ventilatory support, but organs could not be removed while the heart was still beating.

Brain death is legally recognised in Argentina, Brazil, Chile, Colombia, Peru, Uruguay, and Venezuela. It is also legally recognised in Cuba, and the first International Symposium on Brain Death was held in Havana in September 1992. There were representatives from many South American countries, as well as from Europe and the United States.[18] The most useful outcome of the symposium was the very positive response evoked by the recommendation to refer to the condition being discussed as *muerte encefálica* (whole brain death) rather than *muerte cerebral* (with its implication of pathology confined to the cerebral hemispheres.) This first major linguistic hurdle overcome, it became possible to focus more sharply on the different components of *muerte encefálica*. Advocacy of brainstem death got a good hearing, merging with important local work being done on brainstem auditory evoked potentials.[19] In Argentina the recent editorial of a widely read neurological journal bore the title "*Muerte Encefálica, Muerte Cerebral o Muerte Troncal?*" and concluded that 'in the future we will be speaking of death of the brain stem (*muerte troncal*) when referring to what we currently think of as "whole-brain death."'[20] This statement marks a major step forward in Latin American opinion.

In 1982 both brain death and organ transplantation were declared *hallal* (permissible) by the Ulema Commission, the highest religious authority on such matters in Saudi Arabia, and hence throughout the Islamic world.

Turkey (where electroencephalography or angiography must be performed) has now legally accepted brain death.

In Israel, a 1987 regulation issued by the Ministry of Health stated explicitly that brain death was death. It also stressed that irreversible loss of brainstem function was the factual equivalent of brain death. Political and cultural considerations have precluded the regulation becoming law, but as rules issued by the ministry carry legal authority as far as medical matters are concerned, the arrangement has successfully legitimised brain death and the transplantation procedures that it permits, while avoiding a formal Knesset vote on a very sensitive issue. The emphasis on properly documented apnoea secured the endorsement of a body known as the "Council for the Adaptation of Talmudic Doctrine to Recent Advances in Science and Technology."

Little information could be obtained about practice in the former Soviet Union. A law was passed in 1987 permitting the recognition of the brain dead state and the harvesting of organs, but the concept was not widely accepted. The present situation among the various republics is confused. In China, details are scanty. It is known that organ donation takes place from executed prisoners with, allegedly, their consent.[21] These are not, as far as is known, beating heart donors. Evidence has been collected to indicate that ethical standards are low in the methods used to obtain these donations.[22]

The Taiwanese code closely mirrors the United Kingdom code. Neither electroencephalograms or angiograms are required. Taiwanese neurologists have conducted the first ever large prospective study to assess the prognosis of deeply comatose patients on ventilators, when given maximum circulatory support.[23] They concluded that "if strict attention is paid to preconditions and exclusions brainstem death can be reliably diagnosed on clinical grounds alone."

In Japan, organ transplantation from brain dead donors is currently forbidden,[24] although cadaveric donation is legally acceptable. Although the majority of the Japanese medical profession agrees with the concept of "whole brain death" and are very ready to "confirm" it with the use of electroencephography, there is no social consensus on the use of organ donation from such patients. Very interesting papers have been published[25-27] discussing the cultural roots of Japanese attitudes (the "polluting" effect of receiving organs from the dead; the blurring of distinctions between "self" and "non-self," the practice of leaving the problem of whether to recognise brain death as death to the individual choice of relatives, in the name of self determination, etc.)

The reasoning underpinning current practice in Australia and New Zealand is, for us, difficult to understand. Their 1993 Guidelines on the Certification of Brain Death[28] state that "the legal definition of brain death is irreversible cessation of all functions of the brain" and that "the medical means by which this is diagnosed is to demonstrate irreversible loss of consciousness and irreversible loss of brainstem function." The two are, of course, largely synonymous, both because the ascending reticular activating system of the brainstem generates the capacity for consciousness, and because the death of the brainstem is, in the overwhelming majority of cases, the terminal infratentorial repercussion of catastrophic supratentorial events. The guidelines however, object to the use of such terms as "whole brain death" and "brainstem death," objections to the latter centring on the fact that "it cannot be reconciled with the legal definition of death." This seems to be a Catch 22 situation: the desire to remain within the legal framework leads to the pursuit of an unattainable objective. No currently available technique or combination of techniques can ever hope to assess "all functions of the entire brain." In the clinical context of suspected brain death there is a great deal more than isolated cellular activity that simply cannot be evaluated. There is no way of adequately testing, for instance, such important brain functions as those of the thalamus, basal ganglia, or cerebellum. If the irreversible loss of all brain function is the diagnostic target aimed at, we cannot understand the deafening silence concerning the role of electroencephalography, which might have helped a little in the pursuit of this unachievable objective.

The 1987 Canadian Guidelines for the Diagnosis of Brain Death drawn up by the Canadian Congress of Neurological Sciences and endorsed by the Canadian Medical Association, very closely resemble the United Kingdom code.[29] Brain death, it is stated, "can be established by clinical criteria alone." Special tests "can be used to support and in some instances supplement the clinical diagnosis." An updated code was drafted by the congress in 1988, which it was hoped would prove "helpful and sufficient for many years."[30]

The Irish Working Party on brain death, whose members were from the medical and surgical Colleges in Ireland, published a memorandum in 1988.[31] The case for brainstem death was put quite explicitly. The memorandum said "the essential element in brain death is brainstem death. If brainstem function is irreversibly lost, what goes on elsewhere in the brain is immaterial; life cannot return." All signatories to the memorandum were "agreed that the EEG was not necessary for the diagnosis of brainstem death."

The position in the United Kingdom is often misunderstood. Although our code carries considerable moral authority (in the light of its sponsorship in 1974 by the chief medical officer of the Department of Health and Social Security and its endorsement in 1976, 1979, and again in 1995 by the Conference of Medical Royal Colleges and their Faculties), it has no legal or even quasi-legal status. The Department of Health assists its distribution and expects that brainstem testing will be carried out strictly according to its prescriptions. The precise status of the code has never been tested in a court of law. Parliament (which alone makes laws) has not addressed the issue, and there is no case law. A House of Lords Select Committee has considered brainstem death as part of an inquiry on medical ethics and given its tacit support.[32] The advice of the committee, which included doctors and lawyers, was that legislation was not needed.

In the United Kingdom brainstem death has long been accepted as representing death. This clear identification has been reinforced by the updated memorandum from the British Royal Colleges in 1995.[33] This suggested that the term "brainstem death" should replace the term "brain death," and that the definition of death should be the "irreversible loss of the capacity for consciousness, combined with the irreversible loss of the capacity to breathe."

The report of the President's Commission

In July 1981 the President's Commission for the Study of Ethical Problems in Medicine and Biomedical and Behavioural Research submitted a report (*Defining Death*) to the president, congress, and the relevant departments of government.[34] The report accurately described the British criteria and contained the statement that "if the brainstem completely lacks function, the brain as a whole cannot function."

Among the appendices to the report were "*Guidelines for the Determination of Death*" drawn up by a large panel of medical consultants to the Commission.[35] The guidelines emphasised the importance of accurate testing for apnoea. They specifically mention the preoxygenation of the patient, the use of an oxygen and carbon dioxide mixture, disconnection from the ventilator for 10 minutes, and diffusion oxygenation during the period of disconnection. The United Kingdom technique has clearly been taken as a model.

The Commission worked closely with three organisations which had proposed model legislation on the subject: the American Medical Association, the American Bar Association, and the National Conference of Commissioners on Uniform State Laws. These groups endorsed a statute, and the report recommended its adoption by congress for all areas under federal jurisdiction. The proposed statute was to be called the Uniform Determination of Death Act. It states:

"An individual who has sustained either (1) irreversible cessation of circulatory and respiratory functions, or (2) irreversible cessation of all functions of the entire brain, including the brainstem, is dead. A determination of death must be made in accordance with accepted medical standards."

The statute is already law in nearly all states. When all states have endorsed it the unsettling situation where differing statutes have been drawn up by various legislatures will finally come to an end. In 1981 there were seven different patterns of legal statute concerning brain death in 33 states, though many states had no statutes. One could have been declared dead in one state and not in another. A wit once claimed that "the shortest road to resurrection was crossing a state boundary." The taxonomy of these statutes had almost become a study in its own right.

The content of the statute is not entirely satisfactory. The "cessation of all functions of the entire brain" is, quite simply, something that is impossible to determine. No available technique or combination of techniques can ever hope to assess "all functions of the entire brain." The Commission's report correctly states that all functions cannot be taken to include "electrical and metabolic activity at the level of individual cells or even groups of cells," but in the clinical context of suspected brain death there is a great deal more than this (cerebellar and thalamic activity for instance, and the functions of the basal ganglia) that simply cannot be directly evaluated.[36]

The statute will give the impression, at least to a lay public, of seeking to identify "death of the whole brain" rather than "death of the brain as a whole." The medical guidelines accompanying the report make the disingenuous disclaimer that "all functions of the entire brain" means only "those functions that are clinically ascertainable," but the introduction to the report states wisely that "in language as well as content, any legislation ought to make personal sense to lay people." The average lay person does not know that many if not most cerebral functions cannot be clinically tested in the context under discussion. And, if someone in a glass house may be allowed to throw a pebble, our own code has also erred in much the same way when it stated that in brain death "*all* functions of the brain have permanently and irreversibly ceased" (our emphasis). All functions are undoubtedly on the verge of ceasing. And all relevant — that is, brainstem — functions have certainly ceased. But neither of these statements is quite the same as asserting that all brain functions have actually ceased. This seems to be as untestable a proposition in London as it is in Washington. But this very untestability is less relevant to those who equate death with permanent loss of brainstem function (for which there are tests) than for those who insist that the neurological deficit should include all the other intracranial systems (some of which cannot be clinically assessed).

The Uniform Determination of Death Act encountered another type of criticism within the United States itself — namely, that "it contains the most serious flaw that the Commission finds in previous statutes: it provides two independent standards of death without explaining the relationship between them."[37] The same point had been raised over a decade earlier in a detailed critique of the Kansas Statute (the first in the common law world seeking to define death.) Kennedy had then shrewdly emphasised that it was "in no way inspiring of confidence in one's doctor to learn that there are two types of death."[38] The new critics point out that "irreversible cessation of circulatory and respiratory functions" works as a test of death (in the absence of cardiopulmonary support) only because it produces the true standard of death: the irreversible cessation of whole brain function. This approach incorporates the useful distinction between a standard or concept of death and a test for death. Their proposed alternative statute would define death in terms of "irreversible cessation of all functions of the entire brain" and then show how such a state could be ascertained in one of two ways: either by establishing an absence of spontaneous circulation and respiration of adequate duration, or (in the presence of artificial cardiovascular support) by tests specifically directed at brain function. This alternative statute would clearly reconcile the claims of conceptual clarity and of practical relevance. All that would then remain would be to amend all this amendment so that it read "irreversible cessation of brainstem functions" instead of "all functions of the entire brain." This would be more relevant because of the ease and thoroughness with which these functions can be tested, because of the prognostic implications of their loss, and because of the relation of this loss to an acceptable philosophical concept of death. Although the debate continues there are signs that logic and clinical expertise are getting the upper hand. A very recent (1995) document from the American Academy of Neurology[39] seeks to provide guidelines in the form of "practice parameters" for "determining brain death in adults." Brain death is no longer unrealistically perceived as the "irreversible cessation of all functions of the entire brain including the brainstem" but as "the absence of clinical brain function when the proximate cause is known and demonstrably irreversible." An accompanying "special article" states: "the clinical diagnosis of brain death is equivalent to irreversible loss of all brainstem function."[40] The practice parameters point out this is a clinical diagnosis and that "confirmatory" tests are "not mandatory" but just "desirable in patients in whom specific components of clinical testing cannot reliably be evaluated." Bedside experience seems to have reasserted its primacy and led to a belated convergence of British and American practice over a very wide field. Is it too much to hope that within the next few years the appropriate terminological convergence will follow, and that we will then all be using a common verbal currency, referring to brainstem death if that is what we mean?

1 Anonymous. An appraisal of the criteria of cerebral death — a summary statement: a collaborative study. *JAMA* 1977; **237**:982–6.
2 Korein J. Neurology and cerebral death — definitions and differential diagnosis. *Transactions of the American Neurological Association* 1975; **100**:210–2.
3 Walker AE. *Cerebral death*. 2nd ed. Baltimore: Urban and Schwarzenberg, 1981.
4 Pallis C. Brainstem death. In: Braakman R, ed. *Handbook of clinical neurology*. "Head Injury." Amsterdam: Elsevier 1990; **13**:441–96.
5 Smith AJK, Walker AE. Cerebral blood flow and brain metabolism as indicators of cerebral death: a review. *Johns Hopkins Med J* 1973; **133**:107–19.
6 Hughes JR. Guidelines for determination of death. *Neurology* 1982; **32**:682–83.
7 Stuart FP, Veith FJ, Cranford RE. Brain death laws and patterns of consent to remove organs for transplantation from cadavers in the United States and 28 other countries. *Transplantation* 1981; **31**:238–44.
8 Duboust A. Prélèvement d'organes: aspects médico-légaux et techniques. *Revue du Praticien* 1986; **36**:1621–25.
9 Frowein RA, Ganshirt RA, Richard KE, Hamel E, Haupt WF. Kriterien das Hirntodes: 3. Generation. *Anästh Intensivther Notfallmed* 1987; **22**:17–20.
10 Roosen K, Tonn CJ, Burger R, Schlake HP. Diagnosis of Brain Death. *Zentralblatt für Chirurgie* 1992; **117**:632–6.
11 Ciritella P. Brain death: physiopathological and current diagnostic approach. *Minerva Anestesiol* 1993; **59**:505–18.
12 Pallis C. Defining death. *BMJ* 1985; **291**:666–7.
13 Rix BA. Danish Ethics Council rejects brain death as the criterion of death. *J Med Ethics* 1990; **16**:5–7.
14 Pallis C. Return to Elsinore. *J Med Ethics* 1990; **16**:10–13.
15 Chiolero R, Deonna T, Despland PA, *et al.* Directives pour la définition et le diagnostic de la mort. *Bull Méd Suisses* 1983; **64**:808–11.
16 Betschart M. Die Hirntoddiagnose. *Anaesthesist* 1993; **42**:259–69.
17 Pasztor E. New law in Hungary concerning brain death and organ transplantation. *Acta Neurochirurgica* 1990; **105**:84–5.
18 Pallis C. Further thoughts on brainstem death. *Anaesth Intens Care* 1995; **23**:20–3.
19 Machado C, Valdes P, Garcia-Tigera J, *et al.* Brainstem auditory evoked potentials and brain death. *Electroenceph Clin Neurophys* 1991; **80**:392–8.
20 Alvarez F. Muerte Encefálica, Muerte Cerebral o Muerte Troncal? *Boletin Neurologico (Fundacion 'Alfredo Thompson')* 1995; **13**:1–2.
21 Hsieh H, Yu TJ, Yang WC, Chu SS, Lai MK. The gift of life from prisoners sentenced to death. Preliminary report. *Transplantation Proceedings* 1992; **24**:1335–6.
22 Organ procurement and judicial execution in China. *Human Rights Watch/Asia* 1994 **6**:2–39.
23 Hung T P, Chen S T. Prognosis of deeply comatose patients on ventilators. *J Neurol Neurosurg Psychiat* 1995 **58**:75–80.
24 Igata A. Problems in brain death. *Asian Medical Journal* 1991; **34**:607–13.
25 Bai K. The definition of death: the Japanese attitude and experience. *Transpl Proc* 1990; **22**:991–2.
26 Namihira E. Shinto concepts concerning the dead human body. *Transpl Proc* 1990; **22**:940–1.
27 Ohnuki-Tierney E. Brain death and organ transplantation: cultural bases of modern technology. *Current Anthropology* 1994; **35**:233–54.
28 *Statement and guidelines on brain death and organ donation*. Australian and New Zealand Intensive Care Society, 1993.
29 Canadian Medical Association. Guidelines for the diagnosis of brain death. *Can Med Assoc J* 1987; **136**:200A–200B.
30 Canadian Congress Committee on Brain Death. Death and brain death: a new formulation for Canadian medicine. *Can Med Assoc J* 1988; **138**:405–6.
31 Irish Working Party on brain death. Memorandum on brain death. *Ir Med J* 1988; **81**:42–5.
32 House of Lords Select Committee on medical ethics. *Report*. London: HMSO, 1993. *HL Paper 21–1*. 1:70.
33 Working Group of Conference of Medical Royal Colleges and their Faculties in the United Kingdom. The criteria for the diagnosis of brainstem death. *J Roy Coll Phys (Lond)* 1995; **29**:381–2.
34 President's Commision for the Study of Ethical Problems in Medicine and Behavioural Research. *Defining death: medical, legal and ethical issues in the determination of death*. Washington, DC: US Government Printing Office, 1981.
35 Medical Consultants on the diagnosis of death to the President's Commission for the Study of Ethical Problems in Medicine and Behavioural Research. Guidelines for the determination of death. *JAMA* 1981; **246**:2185–6.
36 Pallis CA, Prior PF. Guidelines for the determination of death. *Neurology* 1983; **33**:251–2.
37 Bernat JL, Culver CM, Gert B. Defining death in theory and practice. *Hastings Center Report* 1982; **12**:Feb.
38 Kennedy IM. The Kansas statute on death — an appraisal. *N Engl J Med* 1971; **285**:946–50.
39 American Academy of Neurology. Practice parameters for determining brain death in adults. *Neurology* 1995; **45**:1012–14.
40 Widjicks EFM. Determining brain death in adults. *Neurology* 1995; **45**:1003–11.

10 THE ORGAN DONOR AND DONOR MAINTENANCE

It must constantly be borne in mind that consideration for organ donation *always* comes second to basic medical management. Initially the assumption should be that the patient will survive, and all efforts must be directed to that end.

The scope of transplantation can be seen from the box. Since the beginning of transplant surgery, dead patients have been by far the largest source of transplantable organs, but in many countries the donation of a kidney from a live, usually related person is fairly commonplace. It may in fact be the only source if cultural problems make donation from brain dead patients difficult or impossible. Live donation may, however, lead to difficulties. There are not infrequently psychological problems between live donor and recipient, especially within a family group. Some surgeons are reluctant to remove a normal kidney from a donor, fearing the loss of the other through accident or disease. In Japan because of cultural problems live donation is restricted to hepatic segments for liver failure. The sale of organs, reprehensible though it is, has been justified as a useful source of cash in low income groups. Criminal elements may attempt to manipulate such a market.

There are three other sources of donor organs which are currently being assessed.

Scope of transplantation

Heart	Lungs
Kidney	Liver
Pancreas	Cornea
Skin	Cortical bone
Heart valves	Bone marrow

Elective ventilation

Many patients who may otherwise be fit, die on medical wards of lethal intracerebral lesions.[1] If a patient is in the terminal stages of an acute cerebral catastrophe — massive stroke or subarachnoid haemorrhage for instance — and, with the agreement of the relatives, is taken into an intensive care unit, the issue of "elective ventilation" will arise. This implies that the patient is ventilated and managed in the unit until the criteria of brainstem death are met and organ retrieval can be arranged.

Elective ventilation poses many problems — the logistics of airway management and transfer to an intensive care unit, the need for an understanding and sympathetic approach to relatives, and sufficient intensive care unit resources not to make the donor a burden on an overstretched unit. Protocols have to be watertight and beyond reproach.[2] Elective ventilation also raises the spectre of a patient on a ventilator, presumed to be evolving towards terminal apnoea, beginning after a few hours to breathe on his or her own. This has been reported and presumably reflects the reduction of raised intracranial pressure induced by artificial ventilation. Although these patients rarely survive more than a few hours, they may occasionally end up in a persistent vegetative state and thereby cause enormous distress to relatives and nursing staff. In England, the practice is currently (1994) discouraged by the government, who have apparently accepted legal advice that as the treatment is not directly for the patient's benefit it may not be lawful. A recent extended discussion of this point in the *BMJ* has shown that however logical the basic premise behind elective ventilation, there are still great problems ethically, legally, financially, and logistically.[3] In many parts of the United States the Pittsburgh protocol governs the use of organs from patients who have decided to forego life prolonging treatment. It is instituted only after discussions with the patient (when possible), relatives, and other physicians.[4] Procurement of organs does not begin until after "the irreversible cessation of cardiopulmonary function" in the operating room. Arguments still rage about the legal and moral place of such a protocol.[5]

Retrieval from accident and emergency departments

If a patient arrives in an accident and emergency department and dies on arrival or shortly after, the kidneys can be maintained for retrieval by intra-aortic cooling.[6] A special catheter is inserted into the aorta via the femoral artery. This catheter has a double balloon on the end and is sited within the aorta with one balloon above and one below the origin of the renal arteries. Cold perfusate can then be instilled through the catheter to flush out and cool down the kidneys, which can then be retrieved in a fairly leisurely manner. Needless to say, this requires great tact in approaching relatives and good organisation to enable speedy retrieval. It can realistically be done only in hospitals with renal teams close at hand and able to mobilise quickly. It has proved to be a workable method and source under these circumstances. Other organs such as corneas, bone, and skin could of course be retrieved without haste.

Cadaver retrieval

In some units where there is a major shortage of kidneys to transplant the use of kidneys retrieved within a few hours of death has been tried. The results are, on the whole, not as good as those from carefully retrieved and matched donations, but reports from New York,[6] London,[7] Leicester,[8] and the Netherlands[9] show that kidneys from donors whose hearts are not beating, taken within a very short time of cessation of cardiopulmonary function, can survive for one year in 50% to 76% of cases. It would seem that the method is sufficiently worthwhile to make it acceptable in times of acute shortage. It needs a committed team, strict protocols, and close proximity to a transplant unit. Its shortcomings are a higher incidence of delayed graft function and an associated increased length of hospital stay.

The beating heart donor

Great disquiet has been expressed by some physicians (and some lay ethicists) over the whole concept of "brain death" and of the "beating heart donor."[10] [11] They regard the fact that the heart is still beating as implying that the patient may still be alive. Such worries, expressed publicly, do great disservice to transplantation as a whole. Nearly all rational people accept the concept of brainstem death when it is explained in an understandable fashion. All neurologists, to our knowledge, would today accept the proposition that the death of an individual can be diagnosed on neurological grounds, even if the heart is artificially kept going through the provision of artificial ventilation.

Those opposed to the concept of brainstem death find it difficult to accept the dual logic that death of the brainstem means "death of the brain as a whole" and hence inevitably of the patient and that organs are best retrieved (and make more successful grafts) if they continue to be perfused until as close to the time of retrieval as possible. The requirement for a "beating heart donor" applies only to those organs particularly vulnerable to hypoxia — the heart, liver, and pancreas. The kidneys are somewhat less rigorous in their requirements in this respect and can be removed very soon after cessation of the heart beat. Other organs can be taken almost at leisure.

Anaesthesia for retrieval

Despite the death of the brainstem, spinal reflexes may still be present and interfere with the task of retrieval. Organ donors should receive anaesthesia in exactly the same way as a sentient patient. The occurrence of changes in blood pressure or muscular reactions to surgical manoeuvres do not imply the existence of continuing brainstem activity. Any anaesthetist who has had dealings with tetraplegic patients has experienced the fluctuations in cardiovascular activity that can occur when surgical stimuli are applied below the level of the lesion. The "isolated" spinal cord (divided above the sympathetic outflow) has a considerable reflex repertoire and can play a role for a while in the maintenance of blood pressure. Adequate anaesthesia should also allay any fears of residual sentience.

Intensive care management of the organ donor

All potential "beating heart" donors must be managed in an intensive care unit. The major physiological changes associated with brain death mean that only here can adequate medical and nursing management of cardiorespiratory and other problems with suitable monitoring be undertaken.[12-16] It is unlikely that the duration of management will exceed 72 hours.

It is also vital that the unit concerned has a close working relationship with its local transplant unit and is able to call on them for advice at any time. The *direct* involvement of the transplant unit begins only when the first set of tests for brainstem death yields positive results and agreement for donation has been reached. There should be full documentation in the unit of the necessary procedures and protocols to be followed.

General management

Routine monitoring
Ventilation
Fluid management
Cardiovascular management
Thermoregulation
Infection control
Endocrine disturbances
Spinal reflexes

Monitoring

Minimum requirements are hourly measurement of temperature, pulse, blood pressure, urine output, and electrocardiographic monitoring. The use of arterial and central venous lines may produce risks of infection but is necessary to monitor haemodynamic states accurately and to carry out serial blood gas estimations and other investigations. If a patient arrives in a unit with lines in situ it is probably wise to remove them and replace them under strict aseptic conditions unless it is known for certain that they have been initially placed under such conditions. The use of pulmonary artery (Swan-Ganz) catheters is less certain. The patient who is so unstable as to need such monitoring may well be unsuitable as a donor, but most cardiac transplant surgeons feel that optimisation of cardiac and circulatory function requires the use of a Swan-Ganz catheter.[16]

Ventilation

Tidal volumes
Airway pressures
Inspired oxygen concentrations
Blood gases:
- Pao_2: >10 kPa
- $Paco_2$: 4–4.5 kPa

Ventilation

The essential requirements here are that we maintain an arterial Pao_2 above 10 kPa and a $Paco_2$ around 4 kPa. These will maintain good organ oxygenation and minimise respiratory acidosis. They will also prevent further cerebral oedema which might detrimentally affect brainstem function. Administration of supplementary oxygen may well be necessary and should not be restricted. The theoretical damage that may occur to the lung from high concentrations of oxygen is unlikely in the three or four days that are the usual limits of maintenance of an organ donor. If high concentrations are needed from the start the lungs are probably too badly damaged to be suitable for donation. Neurogenic pulmonary oedema may occur. Fluid balance should be carefully monitored to prevent fluid overload and oedema. Needless to say the nursing management of tracheal and pharyngeal toilet must be impeccable.

Fluid management

Intravenous only
(hourly urine output + 20 ml/hour insensible loss + nasogastric aspirate + other losses)

Plasma expanders for falls in blood pressure

Correct changes in electrolytes (K^+, Na^+, Mg^{++}, Ca^{++}, PO_4^-)

Fluid management

Fluids must only be given intravenously. A low to normal fluid intake should be aimed at, say 30 ml/kg in 24 hours. The best way is to replace hourly urine output plus 500 ml for 24 hours insensible loss. To this must be added nasogastric aspirate and any blood loss. We use 4% dextrose in 0.18% saline for urine volume replacement and appropriate fluid such as blood or plasma expanders for other losses. Electrolyte balance is vital. Metabolic acidosis must be watched for and may be caused by low cardiac output or hormonal imbalances. Potassium and sodium concentrations must be maintained with appropriate fluids. Up to 20 mmol potassium an hour may be used to keep concentrations normal. A minimum urine output of 1–3 ml/kg/hour should be aimed for, and diabetes insipidus should be treated with desmopressin 0.5–2 µg intraveneously 8–12 hourly, repeated as required, to keep urine output around 100 ml hour. Dosage of desmopressin should not be excessive as it may contribute to renal shutdown. It is also important to watch concentrations of other electrolytes such as calcium, magnesium, and phosphate and maintain serum concentrations by appropriate treatment.

The organ donor and donor maintenance

Cardiovascular management

The mainstay of treatment is careful correction of hypovolaemia and the maintenance of adequate cardiac output. The simplest clinical signs of adequate perfusion are a warm periphery and a good urine output. A challenge bolus of 500 ml of plasma expander will demonstrate whether a low cardiac or urine output is due to hypovolaemia. Adequate central venous pressures should be maintained at or somewhat above 10 cm H_2O.

Blood flow is more important than a "normal" blood pressure, but a working pressure of 90 mm Hg or more is preferred to maintain organ perfusion. The liver is sensitive to ischaemic damage if the perfusion pressure is less than 70 mm Hg, as is the pancreas. Some units reduce the packed cell volume to around 0.35 to maintain good flow.

Cardiac arrhythmias may indicate a metabolic problem or extension of the cerebral insult. Tachyarrhythmias are common, and bradycardia may indicate progressive coning. Atropine will not cause tachycardia in patients with a dead brainstem, in whom the vagus is out of action.

The use of inotropes to maintain adequate cardiac output and perfusion may be necessary if cardiac output does not respond to fluid treatment alone. It should be remembered that some of them have the potential for increasing myocardial oxygen consumption and increasing the incidence of renal tubular necrosis.

The most usual initial inotrope is dopamine. In doses of less than 5 µg/kg/min it may improve renal perfusion and urine output. Above this dose it will have an increasing tendency to cause tachycardia, renal vasoconstriction, and tubular necrosis. To increase cardiac output we can use dobutamine in doses of 2.5–10 µg kg/min. If there is poor urine output with apparently adequate peripheral perfusion mannitol may be used to maintain a diuresis. The use of adrenergic agents such as adrenaline is increasing, but it is uncertain whether they have deleterious effects on renal circulation and whether they may increase myocardial oxygen consumption. If drug doses have to be large and continually increased it is possible the heart will not be suitable for donation. If pulmonary artery catheters are being used the cardiac index should be maintained at a level consonant with the patient's weight.

Vasopressin is used in many units to improve cardiac output and is effective for this purpose, in doses of 1–4 units/hr.[15] It seems to reduce the overall dose of catecholamines required. It may, however, impair renal function if the dose becomes too large.

Persistent hypertension may be treated with vasodilators such as hydralazine. Experimentally, β blockers have been used, and probably the short acting β blocker esmolol will be of value.

Thermoregulation

Core temperature should be monitored closely on a continuous basis with a rectal probe. A core temperature above 35°C is imperative for correct performance of tests for brainstem death. Hyperpyrexia, although uncommon, normally settles spontaneously. It may be treated by physical cooling. It is better not to give antipyretics such as aspirin or paracetamol because of any potential deleterious effects on renal or hepatic function. We must not forget that pyrexia may also indicate infection, the cause of which must be sought and treated vigorously.

Hypothermia is very common and is managed by active warming with warming blankets and by ensuring that as far as is possible all intravenous fluids are warmed. All inspired gases should also be warmed and humidified.

Infection

A high degree of alertness for major infection is important as its presence, and especially septicaemia, can drastically alter a patient's donor status. All lines and catheters must be inserted aseptically, and meticulous nursing care of dressings and wounds is vital. Chest infections can be minimised by the presence of a properly inflated endotracheal cuff to prevent aspiration, by sterile tracheal toilet, and by adequate physiotherapy. Samples of urine, sputum, and other potentially infected material should be sent for culture daily. Any pyrexial episodes demand serial blood cultures. Should they be positive

---

Cardiovascular management

Correct hypovolaemia
Aim for good perfusion
Working blood pressure > 90 mm Hg
Adequate central venous pressure around 10 cm H_2O
Maintain cardiac output
Inotropes:
- Dobutamine: 2.5–10 µg/kg/min
- Dopamine: up to 5 µg/kg/min
- Adrenaline

Vasopressin

Thermoregulation

Core temperature at least 35°C
Warm all fluids and inspired gases
Active warming of patients
Pyrexia may mean infection. Seek and treat
Febrile patients may need active cooling

Infection

Meticulous nursing care
All lines and catheters inserted aseptically
Pyrexia ⇒ blood cultures (if positive remove all lines)
Physiotherapy to keep chest clear
Daily urine/sputum culture
Prophylactic antibiotics (according to local transplant team protocols)

the infection must be treated by removal of all lines and vigorous treatment with antibiotics. Lines may then be reinserted aseptically. Transplant teams have their own protocols for prophylactic antibiotics, and it is advisable to know what your local team prefers.

Endocrine disturbances

There is growing evidence that giving intravenous tri-iodothyronine (T3) can prevent and even reverse many of the metabolic results of brainstem death and that it will diminish anaerobic cellular metabolism and its associated metabolic acidosis and reduce the need for bicarbonate and inotropic support.[15][16] The doses suggested are a bolus of 4 µg, followed by an infusion of 4 µg/hr. Any adrenal suppression can be treated with intravenous hydrocortisone hourly until the patient is stable, then four hourly. If hyperglycaemia occurs insulin may be necessary. None of these interventions should negate testing for brainstem death provided hyperglycaemia and hypoglycaemia are avoided. A combined infusion of T3, cortisol, and insulin has been claimed to improve haemodynamics, reverse acidosis, and improve retrieval rates and graft function.[15][16] There is more work to be done on this.

Spinal reflexes

If haemodynamic effects and reflex limb movements due to unregulated spinal activity are suspected, the first can be moderated by the use of intravenous opiates, and any major muscle activity may need treatment with muscle relaxants. It is *vital* that these be stopped well before any tests for brainstem death. The presence of limb reflexes will be sufficient to establish that neuromuscular blockade is no longer a factor that might impede testing.

Endocrine problems

Hyperglycaemia ⇒ insulin infusion
Hypoglycaemia ⇒ dextrose infusion
Diabetes insipidus ⇒ desmopressin
Adrenal suppression ⇒ hydrocortisone

Information for the transplant team

Age, sex, height, approximate weight
History of the acute illness and sites of injury
Time of intubation
Medical progress since admission
Previous medical history
Current condition (urine output, etc)
Current medication including inotropes
Current haemoglobin, white cell count, U&E, CXR, electrocardiogram, bacteriology

---

The coordinators, the relatives, and the nursing staff

Once the diagnosis is established and consent is obtained the transplant coordinator can become active. He or she will arrange all retrieval and disposal of organs as well as the various tests necessary to establish compatibility and look for infective problems such as hepatitis or AIDS. Coordinators will need a great deal of information about the patient. The staff in the intensive care unit should liaise with them throughout the retrieval period.

It is commonly found that some nursing staff may be greatly upset by the circumstances surrounding organ donation and the cessation of treatment. This is especially so if they are new or have strong views on the matter. It is important that frank discussion among the staff takes place about a potential donor and that all have the chance to express their views and fears. The most senior clinician in the unit should take the time to explain all the factors concerned in coming to a decision and should endeavour to carry the nursing staff along, having made that decision. It is also very helpful if all nursing staff have the opportunity to have teaching sessions about organ donation early in their service. This is often best done by the local transplant coordinators, who will generally be the most appropriate people to carry out such instruction.

The spectre of brainstem death can cause intense distress and anxiety to relatives. It is up to the medical and nursing staff to bring them to realise, as tactfully and gently as possible, that the outlook is hopeless.

The question commonly asked is, "Are you going to turn the machine off?" This must be answered honestly and full reasons given. The decision is a medical one, so if relatives ask for ventilation to be continued the doctor has failed to help them understand the situation. Usually, relatives welcome the chance to discuss the matter fully and are relieved to find the decision to discontinue ventilation is not theirs. Once the idea of the irreversibility of the neurological condition and of the inevitability of asystole has been accepted the question of organ donation can be broached.

This should initially come from the most senior clinician involved, preferably one the relatives already know. This cannot be hurried, and time has to be allowed for the relatives to talk it through. After the acceptance of the idea of donation skilled counselling may be needed, and it is here that the nursing staff and transplant coordinators excel. Few doctors have the skills to cope with grieving relatives, and they should make use of their experts, helping only when asked. It is worth always remembering what has been said earlier: that while recipients are always in hurry, donor patients and their relatives *never* are.

1 Salih MAM, Harvey I, Frankel S, Coupe DJ, Webb M, Cripps HA. Potential availablilty of cadaver organs for transplantation. *BMJ* 1991; **302**:1053–5.
2 Feest TJ, Riad HN, Collins CH, Golby MGS, Nicholls AJ, Hameed SN. Protocol for increasing organ donation after cardiovascular death in a district general hospital. *Lancet* 1990; **335**:1133–5.
3 Riad H, Nicholls A. An ethical debate: elective ventilation of potential organ donors. *BMJ* 1995; **310**:714–9.
4 University of Pittsburgh Medical Center. *Policy for the management of terminally ill patients who may become organ donors after death*. Pittsburgh: University of Pittsburgh, 1992.
5 Youngner SJ, Arnold RM. Ethical, psychosocial, and public policy implications of procuring organs from non-heart-beating cadaver donors. *JAMA* 1993; **269**:2769–74.
6 Orloff MS, Reed AI, Erturk E, Kruk R, Paprocki S, Cimbalo CS, *et al*. Non-heart-beating cadaveric organ donation. *Ann Surg* 1994; **4**:578–85.
7 Phillips AO, Snowden SA, Hillis AN, Bewick M. Renal grafts from non-heartbeating donors. *BMJ* 1994; **308**:575–6.
8 Vart K, Veitch PS, Morgan JDT, Kehindi EO, Donelly PK, Bell PRF. Response to organ shortage: kidney retrieval programme using non-heartbeating donors. *BMJ* 1994; **308**:575.
9 Wijnen RMH, Booster MH, Stubenitsky BM, de Boer J, Heineman E, Kootstra G. Outcome of transplantation of non-heart-beating donor kidneys. *Lancet* 1995; **345**:1067–70.
10 Evans DW, Hill DJ. The brain stems of organ donors are not dead. *Catholic Medical Quarterly* 1989;
11 Evans DW, Hill DJ, Gresham G A. Availability of cadaver organs for transplantation. *BMJ* 1991; **303**:312.
12 Power BM, van Heerden PV. The physiological changes associated with brain death — current concepts and implications for treatment of the brain dead organ donor. *Anaesthesia and Intensive Care* 1995; **23**:26–36.
13 Timmins AC, Hinds CJ. Management of the multiple-organ donor. *Current Opinion in Anesthesiology* 1991; **4**:287–92.
14 Darby JM, Stein K, Grenvik A, Stuart SA. Approach to management of the heartbeating 'brain dead' organ donor. *JAMA* 1989; **261**:2222–8.
15 Odom NJ. Organ donation. 1. Management of the multiorgan donor. *BMJ* 1990; **300**:1571–3.
16 Pagano D, Bonser RS, Graham TR. Optimal management of the heart-lung donor. *Br J Hosp Med* 1995; **53**:522–5.
17 Novitzky D, Cooper DKC, Reichart B. Haemodynamic and metabolic responses to hormonal therapy in brain dead potential organ donors. *Transplantation* 1987; **43**:852–4.

INDEX

Index

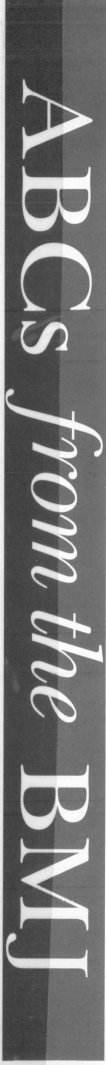
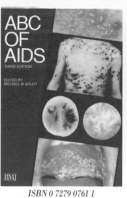

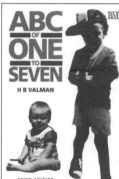
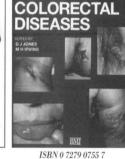
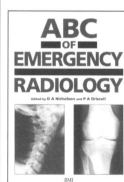
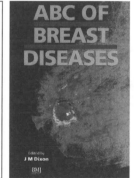
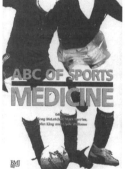
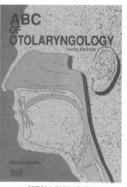
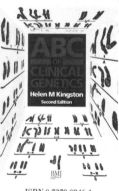
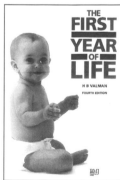
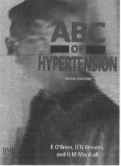

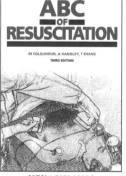
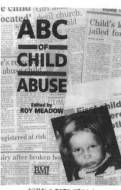